Epilepsy

A Practical Guide to Coping

Dr Ley Sander MD
and
Dr Pam Thompson PhD, AFBPsS

First published in 1989 by
The Crowood Press
Ramsbury, Marlborough
Wiltshire SN8 2HE

British Library Cataloguing in Publication Data

Sander, Ley
Epilepsy,
1. Man. Epilepsy
I. Title   II. Thompson, Pam
616.8'53

ISBN 1 85223 178 5

Acknowledgements

We would like to thank several of our colleagues for their advice and
encouragement. We are particularly indebted to Debbie Cleminson,
Yvonne Hart, Marc McGinty, Mary Moore, Jolyon Oxley and
Simon Shorvon. Special thanks to Suzy Joas and Joseph Miller for
their patience and support. Gratitude must of course be extended to
all the people with epilepsy we have met and from whom we have
learned so much. We dedicate this book to them.

Line illustrations Figs 1–5 by Sharon Perks, Figs 6–9 by
Marc McGinty

Typeset by Photosetting, Yeovil
Printed in Great Britain by
Hillman Printers (Frome) Ltd., Frome, Somerset
Bound by Maclehose & Partners, Portsmouth

Contents

Foreword

This is a unique book. It is written primarily for people with epilepsy and their families, in order to provide information and advice about epilepsy, but is more than a commonplace patient's handbook. The book covers a very wide range of topics, from medical issues such as diagnosis and drug treatment to social issues such as schooling and employment, and practical issues to help sufferers cope with everyday matters. It is authoritative and detailed, yet admirably clear and straightforward, without jargon or condescension.

One reason for its success in achieving its aims is the fact that the book is the combined effort of an experienced doctor and a psychologist. Both Ley Sander and Pam Thompson have devoted the greater part of their professional lives to epilepsy, in one of the largest epilepsy units in the country. They have an unrivalled experience of the problems epilepsy poses. What is also rare is their ability to communicate this experience with such clarity. Although this book is essentially for people with epilepsy and their families, it would also be read with advantage by those involved in the care of people with epilepsy and should be essential reading for social workers, health workers and nurses. This is an important book which will help all of us in our different ways to understand epilepsy better and to cope with this condition in a more informed and competent manner.

Simon D. Shorvon, MA, MD, MRCP
Medical Director, Chalfont Centre for Epilepsy
Senior Lecturer in Neurology, Institute of Neurology and The
National Hospital for Nervous Diseases, Queen Square, London

Introduction

Epilepsy is one of the commonest medical conditions, with at least five people in every 1,000 affected. Worldwide it affects millions of people, and yet no other medical condition seems so misinterpreted and misunderstood. It is one of the oldest recorded medical conditions known to mankind, and was accurately described by Hippocrates, the ancient Greek physician commonly regarded as the father of medicine, over 2,500 years ago. Although he recognised it then as a state of the brain and not the consequence of magical possession, even now epilepsy is misconceived. It is viewed with varying degrees of fear, dread and suspicion and the diagnosis of epilepsy still carries a heavy burden.

For the person with epilepsy, the attacks, which are unpredictable and may occur only occasionally and last only a few moments, are not necessarily the most serious aspect of the condition. The sizeable social stigma attached to epilepsy, its unpredictability and its transient nature may cause considerable demoralisation, frustration and anxiety, not only to the person with seizures but also to family, friends and health care workers. People with epilepsy all too often have to cope not only with their attacks, but with problems in almost every sphere of their day-to-day lives – going to school, making friends, getting a job, choosing a career, and starting a family. These problems should not be underestimated.

In this book we hope to provide some basic information about the condition and, above all, a practical guide to coping with epilepsy. The book is aimed at people with epilepsy, their families, and anyone who has an interest in or contact with them, including social workers, teachers, employers, and colleagues. We feel that correct information and sound advice will help to dissipate some of the myths and misconceptions about the condition and make it easier to cope with.

We have attempted to refrain from medical terms, but some have been unavoidable. When this happens, we try to explain most of them in the text, but for some of them this was not possible. For this reason, at the end of the book there is a small glossary of medical terms. We have used the words 'attacks' and 'fits' interchangeably for all types of epileptic seizures, while the term 'convulsion' has been restricted to generalised tonic clonic seizures (grand mal attacks). We have tried to avoid using 'grand mal' and 'petit mal' as they have now been superseded by other terms, but we have used them on occasion for the sake of clarity.

Ley Sander, Pam Thompson

1
What is Epilepsy?

The word epilepsy is derived from a Greek term which means to possess, to take hold of, to grab, to seize. To the ancient Greeks, epilepsy was a miraculous phenomenon: only the gods could knock down a person, strip him of his reason, make his body thrash around uncontrollably, and afterwards bring him round with no apparent ill effects.

In medical jargon, epilepsy is defined as the occurrence of transient paroxysms of uncontrolled discharges of the nerve tissue of the brain, leading to epileptic attacks. It is necessary for the attacks to be recurrent to constitute epilepsy; by definition, a single attack is not epilepsy. It is fair to say that epilepsy is a term loosely applied to a number of conditions that have in common only a tendency to have epileptic attacks. It is not an illness in its own right, but it is a symptom of many different diseases with different causes, in the same way that headaches can have many different causes.

Epilepsy is a very common medical condition; one in every 150 to 200 persons in the general population has recurrent attacks at some point in time. However, most of these people do not suffer from epilepsy for their whole life. No consistent national or racial differences in the occurrence of epileptic seizures have been found. Seizures may occur at any age but are more common in the first 20 years of life and in the elderly. It has been estimated that more than half of the people developing epilepsy will have had their first attack by the age of 15 years; slightly more males are affected than females.

Epileptic seizures are referred to in many different ways. Fits, turns, attacks, and black-outs are some of the most frequently used terms. Whatever name is used, a seizure is usually a very brief stereotyped event in which an individual's awareness of his surroundings is impaired and behaviour may be altered. Attacks frequently have a sudden onset, are short, and cease spontaneously. A period of drowsiness and confusion may follow. Seizures may take many different forms but are all caused by a sudden disturbance in the normal functioning of the brain.

THE BRAIN

The human brain forms part of the central nervous system, which also includes the spinal cord. The part of the brain of most interest in epilepsy is the cerebrum (the other parts being the brain stem and the cerebellum). It is situated within the skull, separated from the bone by membranes called meninges. Between the meninges and the brain there is a very small space filled with liquid, the cerebrospinal fluid. The brain is a highly complex structure composed of millions and millions of nerve cells, which are called neurones. These cells are ultimately responsible for almost all the functions of our body including movement, posture, memory, emotions, awareness, perception, and so on, and they are distributed throughout the brain. Neurones are very active cells and are in constant need of oxygen in order to function appropriately.

In an over-simplified way, the brain is divided into two halves, called hemispheres. Each hemisphere is further divided into four parts or lobes – a frontal, a temporal, a parietal and an occipital

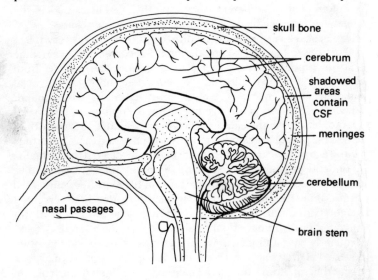

Fig 1   Lateral view of the skull and brain.

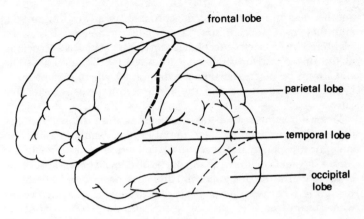

Fig 2   One hemisphere of the brain with its lobes.

lobe. Each lobe is responsible for specific functions of the body or mind. Roughly speaking, the left frontal lobe controls the movement of the right side of the body while the right frontal lobe controls the left side of the body. The parietal lobes control the physical feelings of the body and the occipital lobe the vision. The temporal lobes have a much wider range of functions, including emotion, memory, and perception.

All these nerve cells or neurones which make up the brain are interconnected in a vast and intricate web. Neurones communicate with each other by transmitting impulses. These impulses, or messages, are tiny electrical discharges which are sent and received in an orderly way. Impulses may tell a neurone to act, while at the same time other neurones may be prevented from acting. A neurone can accept or refuse the message, and may subsequently pass it on to

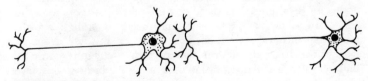

Fig 3   View of two neurones.

9

another neurone. The activity of neurones is usually well organised, and they have mechanisms to regulate themselves. It can be registered by an electroencephalogram (EEG), which is a recording of the tiny electrical discharges produced by the neurones. The EEG may be of great value in establishing whether someone is having epileptic attacks and also in classifying them, as we will see later.

When for some reason the usual organisation is disrupted and nerve cells start sending these impulses in a chaotic manner, an epileptic attack may be triggered. All epileptic seizures begin in this way. The precise features of an attack will depend on the area of the brain in which the first abnormal discharge occurs, and whether it spreads to other parts of the brain. The discharge may involve the whole brain from the start, or it may affect only one part of the brain. Sometimes the discharge expands from a small area of the brain to involve the whole brain, sometimes it will be confined to a tiny area. The part of the brain from which the initial abnormal discharge arises is known as the epileptic focus.

Epileptic attacks may be caused by any process which affects the fine balance of the brain. Anyone can have an epileptic attack if the brain is exposed to certain conditions – indeed this is the way an ordinary brain reacts to abnormal circumstances. This is an important concept: *anyone* under the right circumstances can have an epileptic attack. For example, someone who catches an infection of the brain such as meningitis, or someone who suffers a head injury, or who reacts badly to a certain drug, can have one or more epileptic attacks. Not all persons who experience an epileptic attack will go on to have epilepsy, but a few will. Epilepsy is a disorder of the function of the brain itself, which may result from a variety of causes. Despite this, in a significant proportion of people with epileptic seizures no clear cause can be found.

An important point must be made here. In some diseases of other organs, like the kidneys or the liver, the chemical functioning of our body can be altered considerably and epileptic attacks may then result. In some people attacks may occur if addictive drugs, including alcohol, are used in excess, or if such drugs are withdrawn. In small children seizures may occur in response to a high temperature. Any situation that causes the brain to be starved of oxygen may result in seizures. In all these circumstances, even following recurrent epileptic attacks, the person should not be considered as having epilepsy. As soon as the balance of the body returns to normal, these seizures will cease.

TYPES OF EPILEPTIC ATTACK

When epilepsy is mentioned most people tend to think of grand mal attacks, but although convulsions are the commonest of epileptic attacks, they do not all take this form. A few people with epilepsy may have more than one type of attack, but the pattern of attacks tends to remain fairly constant for each individual. It is important for the doctor looking after people with epilepsy to classify the attacks, as this will have implications with regard to the treatment. However, the classification of epilepsy is a contentious issue, and not all doctors agree about the best method.

Epileptic attacks may be classified and grouped in a variety of ways: by their cause, by the age of the person having them, by the area of the brain where the abnormal discharge starts, by their symptoms, or by the types of attacks themselves. The most widely used classification is the so-called International Seizure Classification, which is a scheme for the classification of seizures based on seizure types proposed by the International League against Epilepsy (an international organisation of professionals who specialise in epilepsy). It divides seizures into two main groups according to the area of the brain in which the abnormal discharge originates.

If it involves both sides of the brain simultaneously, the seizures are termed generalised.

If a discharge starts in a localised area of the brain, they are termed partial seizures.

The differentiation between the two groups is based on the EEG and on the symptoms and signs a person has before, during and after an attack. This is why it is so important for the doctor looking after a person with epilepsy to have an eyewitness account as well as details from the person who had the attack.

In generalised attacks no epileptic focus can be found. The whole of the brain is affected by the abnormal discharge at the same time, and this can usually be demonstrated by an EEG. The person having this type of seizure has no warning, but from the very onset will have impairment of consciousness. There are various types of generalised fits. Among the most common generalised epileptic attacks are:

- tonic clonic convulsive attacks;
- typical absence attacks;
- myoclonic jerks.

Generalised tonic clonic convulsions or convulsive attacks were in the past called grand mal attacks and this term is still widely used today outside the medical profession. They are the commonest of all epileptic seizures. In this type of attack, there is no warning whatsoever. The person suddenly goes stiff, falls, and jerks all over, has laboured breathing and salivates. Cyanosis (a blue appearance to the skin), incontinence, and tongue biting may all occur during the attack. The convulsion slows down and ceases after a few minutes and may often be followed by a period of drowsiness, confusion, headache and sleep. It is not uncommon for the person to fall deeply asleep after an attack. This may sometimes be misinterpreted as their still being unconscious. When they wake up they will always have forgotten what has happened. They usually feel tired and they may complain of pains all over the body. Generalised tonic clonic seizures may happen at any time although some young people have them only on awakening, or shortly after (waking epilepsy). Sometimes they may be precipitated by flashing lights (photosensitive seizures), but usually there is no triggering factor.

Typical absence attacks, also known as petit mal, are a much rarer form of generalised seizure. They occur almost exclusively in childhood and early adolescence. The child goes blank and stares, and fluttering of the eyelids and flopping of the head may occur. The attacks last only a few seconds and often go unrecognised. Even the child having these attacks may not notice them.

Another rare form of generalised attack is the so-called myoclonic seizure. This is made up of abrupt, very brief involuntary shock-like jerks, which may involve the whole body, or the arms, or the head. They usually happen in the morning, shortly after waking. They may sometimes cause the person to fall, but recovery is immediate. It should be noted that there are other forms of non-epileptic myoclonic jerks. They occur in a variety of other nerve diseases, and they may also occur in healthy people, particularly when they are just going off to sleep.

There are several other types of generalised attacks but they are very rare indeed, accounting for less than 1 per cent of the epileptic attacks seen in the general population. They usually occur in the course of some forms of severe epilepsy, starting in early childhood. One example of these is the atonic seizure, also known as the akinetic attack, or drop attack, in which there is a sudden loss of muscle tone of the body and the person collapses to the ground with no convulsions. Recovery afterwards is quick. Another example is the so-called tonic attack, in which there is a sudden increase in the muscle tone of the body and the person becomes rigid and collapses to the ground, usually followed by a quick recovery. Tonic and atonic attacks are often accompanied by severe injury.

Partial, or focal, attacks arise from an epileptic focus. This is the area in which the abnormal discharges occur. The partial nature of the attack can often be identified from the clinical signs present during and after the attack. The EEG trace will often show the location of the focus. Partial seizures are subdivided into three groups:

- simple partial;
- complex partial; and
- partial with secondary generalisation.

The precise nature of an attack depends upon the position of the focus in the brain, and whether the discharges remain localised or spread throughout the brain. For instance, a discharge which starts in that area of the right frontal lobe which controls the movement of the left little finger, provided that it stays localised, will only result in jerking of this finger. However, it may spread to other lobes and even to the whole brain. If it spreads to the area which controls the left arm, then the whole arm may shake or jerk. If it then spreads further to the whole brain, a convulsive attack resembling a generalised tonic clonic seizure may occur. If the epileptic discharge remains localised it is likely that the person will remain aware throughout the attack, as the rest of the brain continues to function normally. If it spreads, consciousness may be impaired. If a person has any warning of his epileptic attacks, this provides evidence for a focal origin of the seizure. Another sign which indicates the focal onset of an attack is the persistence of a symptom after a seizure has finished. For example, a person may experience a temporary weakness of an arm after an attack, or may be unable to speak properly for a while.

Simple partial attacks or focal seizures are attacks in which the epileptic discharge remains localised and in which consciousness is fully preserved. Simple partial attacks on their own are rare and they usually progress to other forms of partial seizure. They occur more often in people whose attacks started late in life rather than in children. What actually happens during a simple partial attack depends on the area in which the discharge occurs and may vary widely from person to person, but will always assume the same form in one person. Localised jerking of a limb or the face, stiffness or twitching of one part of the body, numbness or abnormal sensations of parts of the body, rising sensation or feelings in the stomach, sound, smell or visual sensations are all examples of what may occur during a simple partial attack. It may then cease, or it may progress. If the attack carries on and consciousness becomes altered, it is then called a complex partial seizure. If it evolves further and a convulsive seizure occurs it is then called a secondarily generalised seizure. In attacks which progress, the early part of the fit, in which consciousness is preserved, is called the aura, or warning. This aura gives a clue to the doctor as to the part of the brain in which the focus is located. The warning is usually very short, and sometimes people forget altogether that they had an aura.

Complex partial seizures are seizures which have similar characteristics to simple partial seizures, but they always involve an impairment of consciousness. They may start as a simple partial seizure and then progress, or the person may have alteration of consciousness from the very onset. If the attack begins as a simple partial seizure, the person may then have a warning that the seizure is about to start. Complex partial seizures are a very common form of partial attack. They may present as altered or 'automatic' behaviour. The person may pluck his or her clothes, fiddle with various objects and act in a very confused manner. Lipsmacking or chewing movements, grimacing, undressing, performing aimless activities, and wandering around in a drunken fashion may all occur on their own or in different combinations during complex partial seizures. This type of attack is not always recognised immediately as a seizure, and this can sometimes cause the person having them considerable problems. It is not unheard of for people having complex partial seizures to be diagnosed as having some form of mental disorder, sometimes with unfortunate consequences. As most of the discharges which lead to complex partial seizures start in the temporal lobes, this type of epilepsy is often termed 'temporal lobe epilepsy'. Another term sometimes used is 'psycho-motor seizures'. Complex partial seizures may progress to become full-blown convulsive attacks, and in this case they are called secondarily generalised seizures.

Secondarily generalised attacks are partial seizures, either simple or complex, in which the discharge spreads to the entire brain. The person may have an aura, but this is not always the case. The spread of the discharge can occur so quickly that no features of the localised onset are apparent to the patient or an observer, and in that case only an EEG can then demonstrate that the attack did start from a focus. The involvement of the entire brain leads to a tonic clonic convulsive attack with the same characteristics as a generalised tonic clonic convulsion.

A very small percentage of attacks may remain impossible to classify even after investigations have been carried out. An example of a type of attack which is not always easy to classify is the so-called atypical absence or complex absence, which, like atonic attacks, may occur in the course of severe epilepsy with its onset in childhood. Complex absences are prolonged absence-type attacks with some other feature, such as localised jerks, or twitching.

In addition to classifying epileptic attacks by type, it is important to classify certain types of epilepsies into the so-called epileptic syndromes. A syndrome is a group of symptoms and signs which, when taken together, form the description of an illness. In the case of epilepsy the features which usually make up a syndrome are the type of attack that occurs, the age at the onset of the attacks, and characteristic changes in the EEG. Most of the epileptic syndromes start in childhood or adolescence, and they are sometimes called age-linked epilepsies. One of the reasons for this classification is that some syndromes are best treated by a particular drug. There are also implications for outcome as some syndromes are very benign, and for others the outlook is bleaker. The tests which the doctor is likely to order will vary from syndrome to syndrome; some require no tests at all, while others will require specialised investigations. In addition, the possible complications of the different syndromes are known and the appropriate action may be taken early to avoid them.

The commonest of the epileptic syndromes is the so-called primary generalised epilepsy, also known as idiopathic generalised epilepsy, for which no cause is known. This syndrome accounts for about one-third of all epilepsies, and there is a typical EEG pattern with generalised 'spike and wave' discharges. The onset of the syndrome is usually between the ages of 5 and 15 years, and the outcome is usually very good, as treatment is normally highly effective. The seizure types which may occur in this syndrome are generalised tonic clonic seizures, typical absence seizures and myoclonic seizures, on their own or in different combinations. For instance, some children have frequent absence-type seizures and the occasional early morning generalised tonic clonic convulsion, while others may have only the absences. Waking epilepsy, benign myoclonic epilepsy and childhood and juvenile typical absence-type epilepsy are all patterns of primary generalised epilepsy. There is usually a slightly higher chance of someone in the family of such a sufferer having epilepsy, which suggests that inheritance plays a role.

Another epileptic syndrome is Rolandic epilepsy, also known as benign partial epilepsy of childhood. It is characterised by partial attacks, the EEG showing discharges in a part of the temporal lobe called the Rolandic area. Children with this syndrome usually have only a very few attacks in total, and they tend to occur during the night. The onset is usually between the ages of 4 and 12 years. This syndrome accounts for about 10 to 15 per cent of epilepsy in this age group. It has a very good outcome, and usually does not require treatment. A variety of this syndrome is benign occipital epilepsy, in which the EEG disturbance is in the occipital lobe and these children may present with visual disturbances during the attacks.

Neonatal seizures are attacks occurring in the first four weeks of life. They affect about 1 per cent of babies, and in around one-quarter of cases no cause can be found. In the remaining three-quarters brain damage caused by oxygen deprivation during the delivery, imbalance in the blood chemicals, or occasional rare congenital disorders are responsible for the seizures. These tend to have a poor outcome, as one-quarter of these babies will die within their first year of life, and half will either carry on having seizures into adult life or will have other problems such as mental retardation or spasticity. Only one-quarter will make a full recovery.

Rarer epileptic syndromes include the so-called West syndrome and the Lennox-Gastaut syndrome, which have some common features. Both affect many more boys than girls. Usually the development of the child is normal until the attacks start, but it then becomes impaired. It is believed that the same type of damage to the brain can be responsible for both conditions.

West syndrome was originally described by a doctor in his own baby boy in 1841. It may also be referred to as infantile spasms, Salaam spasms or hypsarrhythmia. The onset is usually around the age of six months, and the child may have suffered some form of identifiable brain damage early in life, but in about one-third of cases no cause can be found. In this syndrome there is a characteristic EEG pattern called hypsarrhythmia, and the attacks consist of sudden generalised jerks, with bending of the head forward, accompanied by flexion of the arms and bending of the knees. These may happen at any time and may occur in clusters. The outcome is gloomy, and the child usually becomes grossly mentally retarded and starts having other seizure types. It does not respond to treatment with conventional anti-epileptic drugs, but in some cases the outcome may be improved if corticosteroids are used early on in the condition.

Lennox-Gastaut syndrome is characterised by multiple seizure types including drop attacks, complex absences, tonic clonic convulsions and myoclonic jerks. It has a characteristic EEG pattern known as 'slow spike and waves' and it is frequently associated with mental retardation. In about half of the cases it appears to start out of the blue, and in the other half causes can be identified. A past history of West syndrome seems to be the commonest identifiable cause. Other causes include brain damage at birth, infections, tumours, and severe head trauma. The syndrome usually affects children between the ages of 1 and 8 years, but sometimes it may start later on. It has a very bleak outcome with regard to seizure control and mental development. Fortunately it is a very rare condition, accounting for perhaps 1 per cent of all new cases of epilepsy, although due to its poor outcome it may account for as much as 10 per cent of people with severe epilepsy.

A special point must be made here about febrile convulsions, which are convulsions occurring in children with a high fever. They are not strictly speaking an epileptic syndrome and are usually a very benign condition, but they must be distinguished from seizures that are triggered by infections of the brain such as meningitis. Febrile convulsions or seizures occur in children between the ages of 1 and 5 years only in the presence of high fever, that is, temperatures of 100°F or more. They are very common, and three or four out of every 100 children will have them. The attacks are usually of the generalised tonic clonic type, but sometimes they may have partial features. The outlook is very good: about two-thirds of children having febrile convulsions will have only one attack, and less than 5 per cent will go on to have epileptic attacks later in life. Children who have very prolonged attacks lasting more than 20–30 minutes, or who previously had signs of brain damage, seem to be particularly at risk of developing epilepsy.

An epileptic attack will almost always stop spontaneously. On very rare occasions, however, attacks may occur in quick succession, without any period of recovery between one attack and the next. This situation is known as status epilepticus. This may occur with any type of seizure, but it is particularly dangerous if status epilepticus involving generalised tonic clonic convulsions occurs. This is one of the few occasions when attacks should be considered an emergency.

2
The Causes of Epilepsy

It has already been said that epileptic seizures may be caused by any process which causes damage to the brain, but despite this, it is not always possible to say why a person has attacks. In about 60 per cent of all cases of epileptic seizures no cause is found. It is very likely that medical knowledge has not yet advanced enough to be able to identify the precise cause behind the attacks. Attacks for which no cause is found are called 'idiopathic' or 'cryptogenic' epilepsy. It is thought that in some people these seizures may be due to an inherited disposition to fits. This basically means that since we all have a tendency to have epileptic attacks, in those people in whom fits actually occur, a lower 'threshold' to seizures may exist, and so a smaller disturbance would still be able to trigger a seizure. This low seizure threshold is thought to be hereditary. It must be emphasised that epilepsy itself is not inherited. What is inherited is either a low threshold, or a disease, of which epilepsy is one of the symptoms.

The outlook for most people with idiopathic epilepsy is very good. Some of the idiopathic epilepsies are very benign and require only a short period of treatment, while others need treatment over a long period of time. They include the so-called primary generalised epilepsies, which have a very characteristic EEG pattern.

The remaining 40 per cent or so of epileptic attacks or seizures occur because there has been some known damage to the brain, either from injury or disease. This is called symptomatic epilepsy. Most symptomatic epilepsy is attributable to head injuries, strokes, brain tumours and infections. A few people may be born with an abnormal brain, others may sustain damage to the brain during birth, and because of this they may have seizures. However, having any of these factors does not necessarily mean that a person will have epilepsy, just that epilepsy is slightly more likely.

The probable cause of the epilepsy depends upon the age of the person: the majority of cases of epilepsy of unknown origin, or of idiopathic epilepsy, commence before the age of 15 years, while the majority of cases of epilepsy with a known cause, or symptomatic epilepsy, start in adulthood. For instance, a cause can be identified in a significant majority of people who start to have attacks after the age of 40 years.

Head trauma is an important cause of symptomatic epileptic attacks. It is often said that it accounts for up to 10 per cent of all cases of epilepsy. The likelihood of developing epilepsy after a head injury depends on the severity of the damage. It is very unusual for seizures to develop unless the injury has caused prolonged loss of consciousness, bleeding inside the head or a skull fracture. The scar in the injured area of the brain will act as an epileptic focus and the seizures will tend to be of the partial type. In the majority of cases attacks start within a year of the injury, and the response to treatment will depend on the severity and the place of the damage in the brain.

Strokes, or brain haemorrhages, are a very important cause of symptomatic epilepsy starting in later life; they are responsible for as many as 50 per cent of cases in this age group. Attacks are almost always partial and, again, usually start within a year of the stroke. Sometimes they may even precede the stroke. It is said that about 15 per cent of people who suffer a stroke will eventually develop epileptic seizures. Attacks due to strokes are relatively easily controlled with tablets.

Tumours which grow in the brain, whether they are benign or malignant, may cause epileptic attacks. Brain tumours usually originate from the brain itself or from the membranes that cover the brain, the meninges, but there may also be 'secondary' tumours which have spread from other parts of the body – from the lungs or breasts for example. Brain tumours are responsible for about 10 per cent of the fits which start after the age of 50 years, and the attacks are always of the partial type. It is not unheard of for epileptic attacks to be the first symptom of a brain tumour. The outlook for a person with epileptic attacks due to a brain tumour is largely dependent on the nature of the tumour.

Epileptic attacks due to infection are rare, but any infection within the skull can cause attacks, and these may continue after the infection has been treated. Epilepsy is a rare complication of meningitis, which is an infection of the membranes that cover the brain. The longer the duration of the disease before treatment, the less effective medication is likely to be and the greater the chances of developing this complication. Seizures are usually focal, and the outlook for total seizure control is in most cases gloomy. Encephalitis, which is an infection of the tissue of the brain itself, usually caused by a virus, may cause epileptic seizures. The attacks are partial in nature and treatment is very difficult. Brain abscess, which is a localised infection of the brain tissue usually caused by germs, is a very rare condition and can often be fatal. Partial epileptic attacks develop in about three-quarters of survivors of brain abscess and are usually very severe and intractable. This is particularly the case with an abscess located in the frontal and temporal lobes.

Another rare cause of epilepsy is injury to the brain of a child sustained during labour. It may be due to direct trauma to the head of the child during the delivery, or to oxygen starvation. The outcome is variable and will depend to a large extent on the severity of the injury. This used to be a common cause of epilepsy in the past, but with the improvements over the past few decades in antenatal care and midwifery, the situation is now very different.

Conditions that affect the child while it is still in the mother's womb may also cause seizures as a result of brain damage. Intrauterine infections are an example of this, as is *Erythroblastosis foetalis*, a rare disease caused by incompatibility between the blood of the foetus and that of the mother.

Epileptic attacks may be a feature of many uncommon hereditary diseases. Tuberous sclerosis and neurofibromatosis are the commonest examples of these. The attacks are partial, and can be very severe.

PRECIPITANTS AND TIMING OF SEIZURES

In the majority of people with epileptic seizures, attacks happen out of the blue, in a totally unpredictable manner. However, in some people there are factors which can trigger fits. If such factors exist and can be identified, measures can be taken to avoid them, thus reducing the likelihood of attacks. Examples of triggers which may occasionally cause seizures in susceptible people are flickering lights, stressful situations, emotional upsets, fear and anger. Other people may have seizures when they take certain drugs or alcohol. The person with epilepsy, their family or friends will often be the ones to notice if any such triggers exist. If it is felt that they do, they should bring this to the attention of the doctor.

A common complaint of some young women having epilepsy is that their seizures get worse around their menstrual period. Hormonal changes and fluid retention are probably responsible for this. In many cases not much can be done about this, but some women will benefit from taking additional tablets in the week preceding the menstrual period.

Seizures occurring during sleep or on awakening are not uncommon. It has been estimated that in about one-third of people with epileptic seizures, attacks only occur during sleep or within one hour of waking. In these people seizures are often triggered by lack of sleep. If this is the case, late nights should be avoided.

A common belief is that seizures are frequently brought on by watching television. In very rare cases this is so, particularly for photosensitive epilepsy. However, it is more often caused by a faulty television screen or poor lighting. There are no reasons to believe that watching a television set which is in good working order, using a computer monitor, or playing computer games should be avoided by the majority of people with epileptic seizures.

3

The Diagnosis of Epilepsy

It can be a difficult task to pinpoint that someone has epilepsy. To start with it has to be demonstrated that the person has a tendency to have recurrent spontaneous epileptic seizures. Yet the one feature that distinguishes epilepsy from other conditions is its unpredictability and its transient nature. For most of the time, it is not there and the examination of a person between attacks is usually completely normal.

The attacks may take a number of different forms, and can thus have many different consequences. If a person starts having attacks or 'funny spells' it is likely that his GP will refer him for a specialist opinion to try to make a diagnosis. This is such an important issue, with so many implications for the person involved, that it is recommended that he should see a specialist. This may be a neurologist in the case of adults, and a paediatrician in the case of children. Elderly people may be referred to a geriatrician.

How does the specialist come to the conclusion that someone is having epileptic seizures? In medical jargon, the diagnosis of epilepsy is essentially clinical; that is, it depends entirely on a reliable account of what happened during the attacks, both from the person involved and from an eyewitness. The doctor may ask for some tests, often including an EEG, but even these may not conclusively confirm or rule out the diagnosis of epilepsy. So it is of major importance that someone who has seen the attacks goes with the person to the doctor. In many cases the diagnosis of epileptic seizures may be straightforward and easy to make, and tests like an EEG may then be ordered only for confirmation. However, on a significant number of occasions there is no witness, or the witness may not have seen the whole episode, and the doctor may have doubts about the nature of the attack. In these cases a series of tests may be ordered to help establish the diagnosis. It is good practice for a doctor to keep an open mind about things; it is a well-known fact that a significant number of people diagnosed as having epilepsy, when properly investigated turn out not to have it. The opposite can also apply here: some people initially thought not to have epilepsy are eventually confirmed as having it.

There are other conditions which cause impairment or loss of consciousness that can sometimes be confused with epilepsy. Another problem is that on some occasions a person may have epileptic seizures only in the presence of a potentially reversible condition, such as a chemical imbalance in the body fluids (for example, low blood sugar), and the doctors will also need to rule this out. However, before ordering any test, the doctor will want to know all the details of the attack or attacks from the person who experienced them and from the eyewitness. (Of course, if it is a small child, the parents will be asked most of the questions.) The following are examples of questions which may be asked:

Was the person who experienced the attack tired, upset, hot, hungry or thirsty?

Had they been previously well? Did they have nausea, dizziness, breathlessness, chest pain or palpitations before the attack?

Had there been any recent drug or alcohol abuse?

Did they have any warning immediately before the attacks – and if so, what was it like?

Do they have any recollection of the attack? If not, what was their first memory afterwards?

Did they fall on the floor, and was there any injury?

Was there any numbness or weakness after the attack?

How many attacks were there in all? Was there only one type of attack, or were there other types of fits?

Have they seen a doctor before for the attacks? If so, what tests did he carry out? Were any drugs prescribed? What did the doctor tell them?

Were there any problems at the time of their birth? Have they ever had any head injuries? Did they ever have any attacks or convulsions with fever as a child?

Does anyone else in the family have attacks of any sort?

The person witnessing the attack may be asked:

What was the person doing at the time the attack started?

What actually happened to the person before, during and after the attack?

How long did the attacks last?

Based on the answers to these questions and a physical examination, the doctor will be in a better position to decide what to do next. He or she may then be satisfied that the person had a seizure. More often, tests will also be needed; these may or may not help in clarifying the situation, and if there is still any doubt about the diagnosis it may be necessary to wait and let time decide – a diagnosis of epilepsy should only be made when there is no doubt.

There are some conditions which are often confused with epileptic attacks, and these all have to be ruled out. The most common of these are faints, heart diseases, stroke, migraine, temper tantrums, and psychogenic seizures.

Faints (known as syncope or vasovagal attacks in medical jargon) are quite common. They happen when, for some reason, there is a rapid drop in blood pressure, so not enough blood gets to the brain. They very often happen when the person is standing up. There is usually a triggering factor, such as anxiety, seeing blood, being frightened, being in a crowded place, being hungry, being hot, or having a bad shock. In older people particularly, fainting may sometimes be caused by a heart problem. Faints are said to be three or four times more common in women than in men. They may resemble epileptic attacks, but there are usually some tell-tale differences. Syncope starts with a feeling of unease, sometimes with blurring of the vision or buzzing in the ears. A person who is fainting falls to the ground gently, and there is usually no injury. Unconsciousness is very brief indeed. The person is usually sweating and pale. Recovery is very quick, and there is no confusion afterwards. Usually nothing needs to be done, but in elderly people it would be recommended that they should have a check-up to make sure that nothing is wrong with their heart.

Migraine is a condition characterised by attacks of intense headache, usually over one side of the head, accompanied by nausea and sensitivity to light. Sometimes other symptoms, such as pins and needles, jerking of the arms or legs, or visual disturbance may occur. The cause of migraine is not known, although some people may have their attacks triggered by a particular factor. Examples of such precipitating factors are stress, emotional problems, and certain foods – cheese, chocolate or red wine, for example. Migrainous attacks start very slowly, and they last much longer than an epileptic attack. They are usually not difficult to differentiate from epilepsy.

A stroke usually happens when the blood supply to a region of the brain is reduced or interrupted by blood clots sticking to the vessels which irrigate that region. This will result in brain damage, and is frequently accompanied by symptoms such as the sudden paralysis of the arm and leg on one side, confusion, or loss of speech. The onset is very sudden, but the recovery is slow. A stroke may leave an area of damage which can later act as an epileptic focus, and this may cause some confusion. Strokes are much more frequent in elderly people than in the young.

Temper tantrums in children can sometimes be confused with seizures. This is particularly true if the tantrum is accompanied by a breath-holding spell. This may cause a very short attack, which may be confused with an epileptic seizure. A good account from a witness usually clarifies matters. Of special importance is what was happening to the child just before the attack.

Psychogenic attacks could be better described as attacks which are not caused by epileptic discharges in the brain. They are not very common in the general population. This type of attack may be triggered by a desire for care and attention, and may be used as a way to manipulate people, in a conscious or subconscious manner. Such attacks almost invariably happen in the presence of other people. Psychogenic attacks (which are also known as pseudo-seizures or hysterical fits) are more variable, and usually more dramatic, than epileptic seizures. Wild movements of the arms and legs are not unusual. The attacks are commoner in women than in men and usually do not respond to anti-epileptic treatment. They can be brought about by anxiety, stress, or pain, and quite often happen in people who also have genuine epileptic attacks, or whose relatives have epilepsy. This can cause considerable difficulties with the diagnosis. Psychogenic attacks may be successfully treated by psychological intervention, but it is sometimes very difficult to make the distinction between true seizures and psychogenic ones.

DIAGNOSTIC TESTS

The doctor looking after the person having the attacks will frequently ask for some tests to be done. These will usually assist the doctor to decide whether the person did have an epileptic seizure or not, and if so, to establish the type of epilepsy, since this has important implications for treatment. The electroencephalogram (EEG) and the brain scan are the commonest of these tests.

The Electroencephalogram (EEG)

For the majority of people with epileptic attacks this is the only test required. The EEG is an invaluable test which should be carried out on almost all people having attacks which are thought to be epileptic. It is a recording of the tiny electrical discharges generated by the neurones, and it is obtained by placing very small metallic pads, usually twenty, to the scalp. These pads are coupled to a graphic device which registers the activity on the paper. In normal circumstances, it takes twenty to thirty minutes to record, and it is a safe and usually pain-free procedure. After having the electrodes attached to the head, the person is asked to lie still on a couch or to sit still in a chair. In persons with epileptic attacks, abnormal discharges of the neurones may be recorded. Epileptic discharges will produce an abnormal recording and certain epileptic syndromes will usually produce patterns which are easily recognised. Some epileptic syndromes, such as 'primary generalised epilepsy', will produce a pattern which is typical of the condition.

People undergoing an EEG recording will be asked to open and close their eyes regularly, and at some point they will usually be asked to breathe deeply for about three minutes. Towards the end of the recording a flashing light may be used, with the person being asked to look directly into it. In a few people this will elicit an abnormal response which might not otherwise be seen. The 'ideal' situation would be for someone to have an attack whilst an EEG was being recorded, but it is very unusual for this to occur.

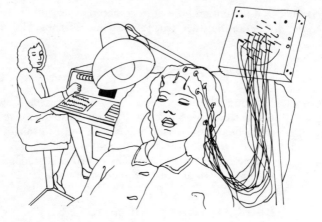

Fig 4   Performing an electroencephalogram (EEG).

Despite the fact that it may be very useful, the EEG does have limitations which should be clearly understood. About 5 per cent of totally normal people have an abnormality in their EEG recording, while 20 per cent of people with epilepsy have a normal EEG. An EEG cannot necessarily, therefore, confirm or refute the diagnosis of an epileptic nature for attacks. The diagnosis of epilepsy must be strongly supported by a bona fide history compatible with seizures. The EEG helps the doctor distinguish between partial and generalised attacks, in locating the focus of an attack, and in assessing the treatment and progress of a person with epilepsy.

As has been said, the chance of recording the discharges of an actual attack during a routine EEG, which usually takes only 20 to 30 minutes, are very slight, and sometimes more sophisticated technology is used for this. Twenty-four-hour EEG monitoring and videotelemetry are examples of this.

Twenty-four-hour monitoring, or ambulatory EEG, allows the activity of the neurones to be recorded for several days, or even weeks. The person has a small number of electrodes, usually eight, attached to his head. These are connected to a small cassette tape recorder, very much like a personal cassette player. The person then goes about his day-to-day life and any abnormal discharge will be recorded. There is a button on the recorder which may be pushed,

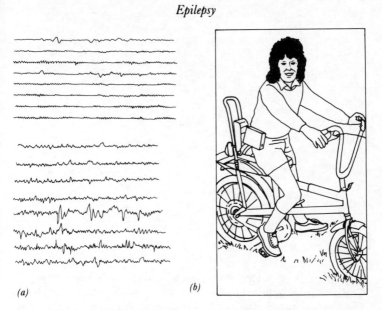

Fig 5 (a) Top: normal EEG recording; bottom: abnormal EEG recording.
(b) Ambulatory EEG monitoring.

either by the person himself or an observer, when the person has an attack. The tapes are later read at the clinic, and any abnormalities identified. This type of recording has a number of uses, and it may be helpful in differentiating real epileptic seizures from psychogenic attacks.

Videotelemetry is a test which uses both videotaping and EEG simultaneously. The person is admitted to a hospital, remains in a room, and is videotaped continuously. EEG electrodes will be attached to the head, but the person will be allowed free movement within the room. The goal is to detect an attack and to record it on the videotape while at the same time obtaining an EEG trace of the fit. This is only helpful in a very few cases, and it is best suited to persons who have very frequent attacks.

Brain Scans

Computerised Tomography (CT) scans are a very valuable test for identifying abnormalities in the structure of the brain. They are

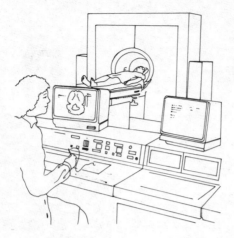

Fig 6 A CT scan being performed.

performed using a special computerised type of X-ray technique. The machine itself looks something like a giant washing machine. The person having the test lies still on a mobile couch, and this moves the head into the scanner itself. X-rays analysed by computer will then show the brain in a considerable amount of detail. The test may detect scar tissue, cysts or abnormal vessels, as well as brain tumours. Not everybody having seizures needs a CT scan, and in over 80 per cent of people it will be normal. The doctor will decide for each individual case whether a scan might be helpful.

With the recent advances in technology, a more advanced breed of scanners, such as the Magnetic Resonance Imaging (MRI) or the Positron Emission Tomography (PET) has evolved. These are very specialised machines, and between them they may identify a great number of lesions or areas of brain damage that could cause epileptic seizures. They are necessary only in a very small number of people and are usually used in situations in which the CT scan was not entirely clear.

Blood Tests

Blood tests are usually required to check the person's general health, and on some rare occasions they may help to exclude a chemical imbalance of the body fluids as a cause for the attacks.

4

Treatment

IN THE EVENT OF ATTACKS

Epileptic attacks are quite common and it is likely that many people will have seen one at some point. When watching, some people have an understandable urge to help the person having the attack. However, there is a great deal of uncertainty about the appropriate response to seizures. So what are the correct things to do, and to avoid doing, if someone is having a seizure?

Generalised convulsive attacks are the commonest type of epileptic seizure. Although they may look frightening, the person having them is not in pain, and will usually have no memory of the attack afterwards. Although knocks and cuts may occur, there is usually no serious injury. The attacks are almost always short-lived, and do not require medical treatment on the spot.

- The person should be made as comfortable as possible, preferably lying down (ease to the floor if sitting). Cushion the head and loosen the collar.

- During the attack, the person should not be moved, unless he or she is in a dangerous place, such as in the road, by a fire or hot radiator, at the top of stairs, or by the side of deep water.

- Do not attempt to open the person's mouth or put anything between the teeth. Do not try to force any medication into the mouth during the attack.

- After the attack has ceased, the person should be rolled on to his or her side. Make sure the mouth and the airway to the lungs is clear of any obstruction, such as dentures or vomit.

- Make sure that there are no injuries which may require medical attention.

- Do not call an ambulance unless there is a serious injury, the seizure lasts more than ten minutes, or several attacks occur one after the other without the person recovering consciousness between them.

Complex partial attacks are usually less dramatic. Alteration of consciousness always occurs, sometimes with involuntary movements, slurring or loss of speech, inappropriate behaviour, automatisms and confusion. Provided several attacks do not occur one after the other, and they are not prolonged (that is, they do not last longer than about twenty minutes), not much needs to be done. During the attack the person should not be restrained, unless he is at risk of hurting himself.

When the seizure is over, some people may experience a period of confusion, while others may sleep. They are often muddled at first and may be unaware of their surroundings, and so it is very important to reassure them during this period of awakening.

In a few cases in which seizures are long-lasting or where they occur one after the other, treatment on the spot may be necessary. This is essential in people who have had status epilepticus in the past. The treatment of choice is Diazepam (valium). It can be administered orally (in between seizures) or rectally. If a doctor is present he may inject Diazepam into a vein. It is usually very effective and should prevent further seizures in the short term. However, it is not useful for the control of seizures in the long term. The doctor who is looking after the person is the best one to advise about the circumstances for use and dose of Diazepam.

THE LONG-TERM TREATMENT OF EPILEPSY

The principal means of long-term treatment for epileptic attacks is drug treatment, and there are several important points which the doctor looking after the person with epilepsy will want to consider in this respect. Starting treatment with a drug is a major event in a person's life, so there should be no doubt that the correct diagnosis has been made. Each individual case should be carefully assessed, as there will be a slightly different situation with each person. Factors the doctor will probably take into account when deciding upon treatment include:

- The number of attacks the person has, and the gap between them.

- The presence of precipitating factors, such as drugs, alcohol, or flashing lights.

- The presence of other medical conditions, especially if neurological or psychiatric.

- The person's willingness to accept the treatment.

- The person's social circumstances.

- The potential toxic effects of the drugs.

Single seizures are not considered to be epilepsy, which is itself defined as the tendency to have *recurrent* attacks. Single seizures do not usually require treatment unless they are associated with a progressive brain disorder, or if there is a clearly abnormal EEG. This only applies to a very few cases, and in the great majority of people the doctor will postpone treatment until a second seizure occurs, which in fact may never happen. If there are long intervals between seizures (over two years, for example), there may still be a case for not starting treatment, but again, each case must be considered on its own merits, and no firm rules can be made. If more than two attacks have occurred, and they were clearly associated with a precipitating factor such as fever or alcohol, treatment should not be necessary. If recurrent seizures are clearly associated with identifiable triggers like alcohol or flashing lights, then steps can be taken to avoid or to minimise their effects. The person's feelings with regard to treatment are also very important and must always be considered. If treatment is to be successful it is essential for the drugs to be taken reliably as prescribed. The advantages of seizure control must always be balanced against the potential harmful effects of drugs.

When the diagnosis of epileptic seizures is beyond doubt, and having established that a person requires treatment and is willing to comply with it, the next question will be: which drug?

THE DRUGS

The aim when starting to treat epilepsy with drugs is to control the attacks with a single drug, using the lowest possible dose and with as few side-effects as can be managed. If the type of the person's seizures is accurately diagnosed, and with the number of drugs currently available, it should be possible to achieve complete control in about 75 to 80 per cent of those having attacks. Sometimes the seizures may not be controlled, or the person may have unnecessary side-effects because the drug used is not the best one for the type of seizures, or it is not being given in the appropriate doses. Some drugs are more effective than others for a certain seizure type, but the effectiveness may differ from person to person. Certain drugs have more side-effects than others, and these too may differ from person to person. It is not surprising, therefore, that in many cases achieving the best result is somewhat a matter of trial and error and it may take the doctor some time to hit on the right drug for a particular person.

There are ten drugs available at the moment which are widely used by doctors in the treatment of epilepsy. In addition, some other drugs are occasionally used, and there are a number of drugs being developed which may become available before very long. The drugs are divided into two groups:

First line drugs, or drugs of choice   These are highly effective for one or other kind of seizure, and are usually the first choice when treatment is started.

Second line drugs   If first line drugs are not satisfactory, a second line drug is used instead of, or in some cases as well as, a first line drug.

Each drug has at least two names. The first one is the generic or chemical name, and the second is the name given by the manufacturer. For instance, carbamazepine is a generic name, and Tegretol is the name used by the maker of the drug, a brand name. If a drug has more than one manufacturer it is likely that each of them will call it by a different name.

Side-Effects

All drugs can produce side-effects and these are usually well known. The person should always be warned about the possibility of them occurring. Side-effects can be divided into three categories:

Allergic reactions   These are rare and usually happen soon after starting the treatment. They occur because the person is sensitive to the drug, and there is no way of knowing this beforehand. Such reactions often take the form of an itchy skin-rash, and they require the drug to be stopped.

Acute dose-related effects   These are the commonest type of side-effect. They are produced by high doses of the drug, and disappear if the dose is reduced or the schedule for taking the medication rearranged. The commonest dose-related side-effect of almost all the drugs is similar: a feeling of drunkenness. People will complain of drowsiness, unsteadiness when walking, dizziness, poor concentration and memory, and slurred speech.

Chronic effects   These are rare, and occur only after the prolonged use of certain drugs. People taking only one drug will usually not suffer from this type of effect, as it tends to affect people taking a combination of drugs. Gum swelling, acne and weight gain are examples of chronic effects. They generally improve when the drug responsible is decreased or stopped.

The table below gives a summary for each of the drugs currently available. Information given includes common side-effects, the type of epilepsy for which the drug is used, and whether it is a first or second line drug. The range of doses, generic and commercial names are also given.

Table 1   Drugs prescribed for epilepsy.

Chemical or generic name:	**Acetazolamide**
Given name:	Diamox
Made by:	Lederle
Available in:	Tablets of 250 and 500mg.
Dosage and frequency:	250–1000mg daily divided into two or three times a day.

Use in epilepsy:	Second line drug occasionally used in combination with other drugs for difficult to control partial seizures and atypical absences.
Other uses:	Its main use is in the eye condition glaucoma.
Side-effects:	Lack of appetite, loss of weight, drowsiness, depression, pins and needles in extremities, joint pains. These are quite rare.

Chemical or generic name:	**Carbamazepine**
Given name:	Tegretol
Made by:	Ciba Geigy
Available in:	Tablets of 100, 200, 400mg, and as a suspension 100mg/5mls.
Dosage and frequency:	Average daily dose range 600–1,800mg for adults; 100–1,000mg for children. Usually taken two or three times daily, higher doses may require four times.
Use in epilepsy:	First line drug for all partial epilepsy. Very effective in some cases of generalised tonic clonic seizures. Ineffective against absences.
Other uses:	Trigeminal neuralgia and some psychiatric disorders.
Side-effects:	Double vision, unsteadiness and nausea may occur initially or if the dose is too high. In a small number of people a skin rash may appear early on in treatment, and requires the drug to be stopped. It may reduce the blood white cell count in some people, but this is only rarely of significance.

Chemical or generic name:	**Clobazam**
Given name:	Frisium
Made by:	Hoechst
Available in:	10mg capsules.
Dosage and frequency:	Average daily dose 10–30mg. Taken once or twice daily.
Use in epilepsy:	Second line drug. Very effective against generalised tonic clonic and partial seizures, but effectiveness may wear off with time. Useful in seizures affecting women during periods.

Other use:	May help anxiety.
Side-effects:	Drowsiness and sedation may occur with higher doses.

Chemical or generic name:	**Clonazepan**
Given name:	Rivotril
Made by:	Roche
Available in:	0.5 and 2mg tablets.
Dosage and frequency:	Average daily dose range 0.5–6mg, divided into two doses.
Use in epilepsy:	Second line drug. Effective against myoclonic seizures, absence and partial seizures, but effectiveness usually wears off with time as tolerance develops.
Other use:	Used for anxiety.
Side-effects:	Drowsiness and sedation are quite common but these may wear off with time. Irritability and mental changes may occur in a few people. Hypersalivation is not uncommon in young children.

Chemical or generic name:	**Diazepam**
Given name:	a) Valium b) Diazemuls c) Stesolid
Made by:	a) Roche b) KabiVitrum c) CP Pharmaceutical
Available in:	a) Injection b) Injection c) Injection and rectal tubes.
Use:	Not used as a regular treatment, only for emergency, and intermittent use. It is the first choice drug for the treatment of status epilepticus and serial seizures. May be given rectally or by injection into a vein.
Other use:	In its tablet form can be used for short treatment periods for anxiety and insomnia.
Side-effects:	It can be quite sedating and in high doses may interfere with breathing.

Chemical or generic name:	**Ethosuximide**
Given name:	a) Zarontin b) Emeside
Made by:	a) Parke Davis b) LAB
Available in:	250mg capsules and syrup, 250mg in 5ml.

Dosage and frequency: Average daily dose range 500–1,500mg in adults, and 250–750mg in children, divided twice or three times daily.

Use: First line drug for absence seizures only.

Side-effects: Stomach upsets, dizziness, drowsiness, headaches, unsteadiness may occur initially or if the dose is too high. In some people it may worsen generalised tonic clonic seizures. Occasionally skin rashes and depression may occur.

Chemical or generic name: **Phenobarbitone**

Given name: a) Gardenal   b) Luminal

Made by: a) May & Baker   b) Winthrop

Available in: 15, 30, 60, 100mg tablets and as 100mg spansule.

Dosage and frequency: Average daily dose range 30–200mg. 5–8mg per kg in children. Once or twice daily.

Use: Second line drug. Effective against tonic clonic attacks, less effective against complex partial and absence seizures.

Side-effects: Tiredness, sedation, lethargy and slowing of mental performance are the commonest side-effects and may occur even in low doses. Allergic skin rashes may occur. Restlessness and depression in the elderly and hyperactivity in children are well-known side-effects of this drug.

Chemical or generic name: **Phenytoin**

Given name: Epanutin

Made by: Parke Davis

Available in: Capsules of 25, 50 and 100mg, chewable tablets of 50mg and as suspension 30mg/5ml.

Dosage and frequency: Average daily dose range 200 – 500mg for adults. In children, 5–8mg per kilogram. Taken once or twice a day.

Use: First line drug for partial seizures and generalised seizures with the exception of absences seizures.

Side-effects:	Drowsiness, unsteadiness, slurred speech may occur if the dose is too high. May cause allergic skin rashes, swelling of lymph glands, hepatitis and lowering of blood calcium in a few people. Coarsening of facial features, overgrowth of gums, and acne may be a problem with prolonged treatment.

Chemical or generic name:	**Primidone**
Given name:	Mysoline
Made by:	ICI
Available in:	250mg tablets and suspension 250mg/5mls.
Dosage and frequency:	Average twice daily dose 500–1,500mg for adults. 20–30mg per kg in children.
Use:	Second line drug. Effective against generalised tonic clonic seizures and all partial seizures. Not effective against absences and myoclonus.
Side-effects:	Primidone is broken down in the body to phenobarbitone, so not surprisingly it has the same side effects as phenobarbitone. Nausea and vomiting may occur on starting treatment, and it is advisable to start treatment in very small doses.

Chemical or generic name:	**Sodium valproate**
Given name:	Epilim
Made by:	Labaz Sanofi
Available in:	100, 200 and 500mg tablets and syrup 200mg/5mls.
Dosage and frequency:	Average daily dose range 600–2,500mg for adults. 20–40mg per kg in children. Once or twice daily.
Use:	First line drug. Highly effective against absence and other generalised seizures. Less effective in partial seizures.
Side-effects:	Drowsiness, irritability, confusion and tremor are the commonest dose-related side-effects. Hair loss and weight gain in some people, but this is usually not catastrophic as it is reversible if the dose is reduced. Liver and pancreas damage are very infrequent complications.

In addition to these drugs, there are other drugs which may very occasionally be used for seizures that prove difficult to control with the regular drugs. Drugs in this category include nitrazepam, nifidipine, allopurinol, ACTH (in infantile spasms). Some other drugs occasionally used in severe epilepsy can only be obtained by special arrangements (i.e. on a 'named patient' basis). They include drugs such as Methsuximide and Sulthiame. Occasionally, people with severe epilepsy might be asked to participate in trials with experimental drugs. At the moment, drugs in this category include Vigabatrin, Lamotrigine and Gabapentin.

People with newly diagnosed epilepsy should be treated with one drug at a time. The chosen drug should be introduced gradually, starting with small doses to minimise side-effects, which are often worse at the start of treatment. It should be gradually increased until either the seizures are controlled or side-effects due to the drug occur. The level of the drug in the blood can be checked, and sometimes this helps the doctor to find the correct dose for a particular person. Most drugs have a recommended range and it is at the top of this range that side-effects are more likely to happen. If the person takes the drug regularly, and has adequate levels of the drug in the blood yet continues to have seizures or side-effects, the doctor will probably slowly change over to another drug.

If complete control of fits cannot be achieved, despite proper and accurate treatment, doctors generally try to keep the drug therapy as simple as possible. This minimises side-effects, reduces chronic toxicity and thereby increases the likelihood that the person will take the tablets regularly. The majority of doctors feel that a combination of drugs is justifiable in only a very few cases, for example if there is inadequate control with a single drug, or in the case of women whose attacks become worse around the time of menstruation, when an additional drug may be required in the week preceding a period.

Regardless of which drug is used, it is essential that it is taken reliably. It is a fact that the single most common cause for treatment failure is people not taking the tablets correctly. Most doctors believe that it is more important for the total daily dose to be taken accurately, rather than the person being too concerned about the exact timing of the doses. Missing a single dose is unlikely to be dangerous or to result in fits. However, stopping treatment suddenly for more than a day or two is dangerous, and may be followed by a number of seizures.

Most other simple medicines can be taken quite safely with antiepileptic tablets. A few drugs, however, may interfere with antiepileptic drugs, causing their level in the blood to increase, and this may lead to intoxication. Antiepileptic drugs themselves tend to make some other drugs less effective. An example of this is the contraceptive pill, and some women with epilepsy who take antiepileptic drugs may have to use a stronger pill. As far as alcohol is concerned, people with epilepsy have traditionally been told to avoid it, but no problems should be encountered if it is taken occasionally and in modest quantities.

An important note: people with epilepsy are exempted from prescription charges for all antiepileptic drugs. More details can be obtained from a person's GP or the local social service office.

STOPPING DRUGS

The decision as to when people should stop taking drugs is a very hard one for the doctor to make. Although some people may require treatment for life, it is often recommended that drugs should be discontinued after a period of three or four years without seizures in the case of adults, and after two years in children. This is a difficult problem, as stopping medication is associated with an increased risk of further attacks. Factors which are usually associated with the successful withdrawal of treatment include:

- primary generalised epilepsy
- absence of other neurological problems
- short duration of epilepsy
- normal EEG

Factors against stopping treatment are:

- epilepsy starting in late life

41

- partial epilepsy
- presence of an additional brain disorder
- long duration of epilepsy
- the presence of an abnormal EEG

In addition, the social circumstances and the willingness of the person to stop treatment should be taken into account. Here again, all cases should be assessed on an individual basis.

If it is decided that the drug should be stopped it should be tapered off over a long time span, as the abrupt withdrawal of treatment may carry a serious risk of seizures returning. In some cases this process may take six to twelve months.

OTHER TREATMENTS

In a few carefully selected people whose seizures are not controlled by tablets and who have an obvious focus, surgery may occasionally be appropriate, and in some cases complete control of seizures may be achieved. The main criterion for selection is the presence of a focus which can be easily reached surgically, without damage being caused to such important areas of the brain as those responsible for memory, speech or movement. If the doctor believes a person with epilepsy may benefit from surgery, extensive investigations will have to be undertaken. On the basis of the results of these tests the doctor should be able to decide whether surgery would be an appropriate treatment. Of course as this procedure involves some risk it has to be discussed in depth at every stage with the person and his or her family.

People with seizures brought on or worsened by emotional stress may find that their attacks are helped by learning such techniques as relaxation (*see* Chapter 6). There is no evidence to suggest that alternative medicine or faith healing have a beneficial effect on the control of seizures. However, people occasionally feel that these measures are of benefit. With the exception of some forms of severe childhood epilepsy which may respond to special diets, there is nothing to suggest that seizures are affected by what is eaten.

WHO TREATS PEOPLE WITH EPILEPSY

In the United Kingdom, the majority of the care of people with epilepsy lies in the hands of the general practitioner. It is usual for people developing epilepsy to be referred to a hospital clinic to see a specialist so that the diagnosis may be confirmed, but further care is normally undertaken by the general practitioner, and in only a few cases will regular follow-up occur at a hospital clinic. However, even people whose epilepsy is mainly supervised by their general practitioner may attend the hospital at infrequent intervals, for example for yearly check-ups.

For people with severe epilepsy special clinics are available in some areas, usually attached to a hospital neurology department. In addition, there are three special assessment centres for people with severe epilepsy. Two are for adults, one situated in York and the other in Chalfont St. Peter (Buckinghamshire), and one for children, situated in Oxford. Two further centres for adults, in London and Cheshire, offer assessment for epilepsy. Addresses for those can be found in Useful Addresses, page 94.

PROGNOSIS

The overall outlook of epileptic seizures is very good. About 75–80 per cent of people experiencing recurrent seizures will eventually become seizure-free, and about half of these will come off drugs successfully. Factors associated with a good outcome include:

- seizures starting in childhood or early teens which are not associated with brain damage

- only one seizure type

- good response to initial treatment

- few or infrequent seizures

- absence of brain lesion

- absence of additional handicap, such as retardation or psychiatric disturbance

The outlook is likely to improve as ongoing research into new drugs progresses, and there are a number of drugs now undergoing trial which appear very promising. Unfortunately, on the other hand, there are some people who will continue to have seizures whatever medication is taken. It is well known that some seizures with a partial onset can be very difficult to control. It is important, nevertheless, that the doctor tries hard to control these attacks using all the available drugs, one by one, and sometimes in combination. The seizures may eventually subside after many months involving numerous changes in the treatment with different drugs at ever-increasing dosages. However, it is equally important that people with severe seizures are not over-treated with medications, as this is likely to produce side-effects which can be more of a problem than the fits themselves. As mentioned earlier, a very few people with seizures which are resistant to all available drugs may benefit from a surgical operation.

People with uncontrolled seizures might have some additional neurological abnormality, although they may not always be obviously handicapped. In some cases, however, the additional abnormalities are the more important factors and often appropriate therapy will be very helpful.

It is very important that it is established quickly if the attacks are going to respond to drug treatment. If it becomes clear that complete control will not be achieved, people with severe seizures and their relatives should be informed by the doctor, to prevent the fruitless search for a drug which does not exist.

Inevitably, some people who continue to have seizures despite medication will look for alternative forms of therapy. Although remedies such as homeopathy, exclusion diets, hypnosis, etc. may benefit some people, they have not been shown to be universally reliable. Provided that conventional medication is not stopped, these treatments are also not likely to do any harm although they can be expensive and inconvenient.

5

A Lifetime with Epilepsy

Epilepsy is more than a medical diagnosis; it can influence many aspects of a person's life. Concern about epilepsy may increase particularly at times of change in a person's life, such as starting school or work, getting married, planning a family, and becoming a parent or grandparent. In this chapter we assess a lifetime, from early childhood to old age, focusing on common life experiences. We will suggest ways of coping with epilepsy and reducing its impact on family life.

One very important point is that people with epilepsy must avoid putting themselves 'on ice' until they grow out of their fits or until a new drug or treatment is developed that will cure them. Many valuable and irreplaceable life experiences can be lost in this way. Epilepsy should not be allowed to take charge of a person's life.

CHILDHOOD

The Early Years

Seizures in babies and young children can be very alarming and distressing. Parents frequently feel their child is dying during an attack, especially when it is first witnessed. A diagnosis of epilepsy at this age can understandably give rise to feelings of disappointment, guilt, and even anger. In the short term, such feelings are often appropriate; however, if they persist they can lead to unhelpful and psychologically damaging coping strategies. These may range from denying the diagnosis of epilepsy to treating a child as if he or she were physically very ill and constantly needing to be watched over and looked after.

The pre-school years are a very important period of development for a child, with major changes occurring physically, mentally and socially. Environmental stimulation during these years plays an important role in this development. During this time a child starts to talk, walk, begins to handle objects and starts to play on his or her own and with others. A young child needs a wide range of activities to develop and consolidate newly learned skills, and missed opportunities are difficult to catch up on at a later stage.

Parents must seriously question whether they are restricting a child's activities because he or she has epilepsy. Are the limitations set really necessary? Young children can benefit greatly from attendance at well-run nurseries and play groups, and having epilepsy should not prevent their taking part. Activities such as playing and sharing with others can take place in nurseries, and other skills essential to later social development can begin to be practised.

During these early years, children begin to test out family rules, learning what is expected of them in the family. The standard set by parents for a child with epilepsy should be the same as for other children in the family. It is important in particular that parents avoid modifying the way they discipline their child because he or she has epilepsy.

Going to School

There was a time when a diagnosis of epilepsy would be a reason for exclusion from school. Fortunately we live in much more enlightened times and children with epilepsy can, do, and should attend ordinary schools. Difficulties may arise at school, but these may be due to factors which are only indirectly related to epilepsy, and their impact can be minimised.

Beginning school can be a stressful time for both family and child. It may be the first occasion that the child has been separated for a significant period of time from the mother. When a child has epilepsy, this may increase parents' feelings of anxiety at their starting school. We recommend openness between parents and school, even if fits are well controlled. If a school is well informed the chance of misunderstandings can be minimised. In order to provide a child's teacher with adequate information, parents themselves must have a good understanding of their child's epilepsy and any implications it may have for school life. It may therefore be helpful for parents to discuss this with their GP or specialist well in advance of the child's first day at school and to gather information that a teacher may need. Teachers will require information which is largely of a practical nature.

In the early school years it is generally the child's form teacher who will need details about the child's epilepsy. However, in later years a larger number of teachers may need to be informed. It is very unlikely that a child will have a fit at school, but if this were to happen the teacher needs to be prepared in order to react with the minimum of fuss and deal effectively with the fit. A teacher will need to know what the fits are like, and how best to treat them. Parents are the people who can provide this information as they are likely to be the only individuals to have witnessed the child's fits. During the attack the teacher will also be in a position to reassure classmates, and help them from an early stage develop a positive attitude towards epilepsy.

A teacher needs to know not only how to handle a fit calmly, but also to know of the importance of providing an accurate description of the attack. This information can be valuable when treatment decisions are being made. A child's first fit may occur at school, and understandably this may be a distressing time for parents. Once a diagnosis of epilepsy has been established, then openness between parents, teachers and the child's doctor is vital.

It is important that every child develops a positive self-concept. This refers to the way they see themselves (self-image) and the way they assess themselves (self-esteem). A child who has a positive self-image will be an individual who is confident and happy. The development of the child's self-image will be greatly influenced by parents' and teachers' expectations of them. A misconception frequently held is that a child with epilepsy should not be pushed academically as this will cause stress and may result in an increase in seizures. Such a lowering of expectations can lead to the child actually believing him or herself less capable and in this way such expectations can become self-fulfilling prophecies. Teachers are trained to develop each child's potential to the highest level, and this should be the goal for the child with epilepsy. A sensitive teacher, while being aware of a child's seizure condition, will not treat the pupil differently, by letting him miss class tests or field trips.

Normal school life involves participation in a wide range of activities. For children who are not academic high-flyers, sport may offer an area in which they can succeed. Blanket bans on such activities for pupils with epilepsy are unwarranted, and most sporting activities will be suitable if appropriate supervision is given. Indeed, boredom aroused in a child from non-participation can be associated with an increase in attacks.

Most concern is usually raised about swimming. Learning to swim is a useful skill which could be life-saving in the event of an accident in the water. Children who are rather awkward and clumsy on land often find their co-ordination improves in the water. The risk of drowning due to an epileptic fit is low, but some extra cover may be necessary at school. A responsible adult such as a school teacher, together with the swimming pool attendant, can keep an eye on a child and take appropriate action in the unlikely event of a fit. Some schools adopt a pairing system, where weaker swimmers are paired with stronger swimmers, and this can be a useful set-up if a member of the class has epilepsy. It has been suggested that the child with epilepsy should wear a distinguishable swimming hat. We feel, however, that this may make the child very self-conscious and 'different' from his classmates.

Other sports such as hockey, football, cricket, tennis and athletics can be undertaken by a child with epilepsy. Some schools offer a very wide range of activities, including water sports and horse riding. These are generally safe for the child with epilepsy, given that accepted safety precautions are taken (hard hat for horse riding, life jacket for water sports and of course the ability to swim). Subaqua, however, is probably not advisable if the child has epilepsy. A wide range of sporting activities at school should also be supplemented by activities outside school hours. Membership of clubs and the use of other leisure facilities should be pursued.

A child who is treated differently may run the risk of becoming rejected by his or her classmates. This situation needs to be avoided, since reactions from and treatment by other children are obviously vitally important in the building of a positive self-image. A child needs to have a clear understanding of his or her epilepsy, which should be updated when necessary. The appropriate reaction to a fit by the class teacher as suggested earlier can also reduce negative attitudes in others. In addition, if a child does have a fit at school, teachers now have at their disposal a wide range of materials to teach even very young children about epilepsy, thus avoiding the ignorance that can lead to prejudices developing.

It is essential to minimise time lost from school, which can arise in two main ways. Firstly, if a child has a fit at school he may be sent home to recover. If this occurs early in the morning, then a whole day may be lost from school. Recovery from a fit is generally quick, and within a short period a child should be ready to resume class activities. A properly informed teacher would prevent loss of school time due to fits. Secondly, a child may need to attend clinic appointments perhaps once or twice a year for their epilepsy to be monitored. This could result in significant time off school, but this may be avoided by arranging appointments during half-term or school holidays. Most children find that there are some subjects they enjoy at school and others they dislike, perhaps because they find them difficult. Children may welcome clinic appointments and see them as a way of getting out of disliked subjects. The more frequently a child misses classes, the greater the likelihood that he or she will fall further behind and find it difficult to catch up.

An understandable worry of parents and teacher is whether the epilepsy or the drugs will cause learning difficulties. If epilepsy is treated appropriately, with regular monitoring, significant learning difficulties should not occur, particularly if appropriate expectations exist about the child's capabilities and if time off school is minimised. Where fits are frequent they can have a disruptive effect on education. Research suggests that this is more likely to happen if the child has fits that originate in the temporal lobes in the brain. This part of the brain, as has already been mentioned, is very important for learning and memory. If a child's seizures arise in the temporal lobes and attacks are not well controlled, then some learning difficulties may be experienced at school. If a child is experiencing very frequent but small attacks such as absences, these can also disrupt his or her ability to attend in class. These types of attacks can go undetected, and the teacher may not realise that a child is getting a very fragmented picture of the lessons. Fortunately, the drugs available to treat epilepsy have greatly improved over the years, and many of the newer compounds have less influence on school performance than older drugs.

If the teacher knows a child has epilepsy, he or she is in a position to evaluate whether a child is falling behind in certain subjects. If the teachers are concerned that this is happening, then they should discuss it with the parents, and appropriate action can be taken.

This may initially require a re-evaluation of the child's attacks, and with a modification of treatment seizure control may improve, so that the impact of epilepsy on school work is reduced.

An allied concern of parents and teachers is whether epilepsy or the drugs taken can cause behaviour problems. Once again the general answer is that they do not, and where problems arise this is often through factors not directly related to the fits. If a teacher is concerned about behaviour problems, and particularly if he thinks that a particular problem is interfering with learning, discussion with the parents is recommended. A description of changes in the child's behaviour should be provided for the doctor on the next clinic visit. If the behaviour is not thought to be because of any treatment factor or decrease in seizure control, then difficult behaviour should be tackled in the same way as similar behaviour occurring in children without epilepsy. Appropriate discipline for the child with epilepsy is essential, and reprimands will not bring on a fit. Behaviour problems are likely to become more entrenched if a child learns that he is not being so severely punished as other children for misdemeanours. It is essential that both the school and the home have the same approach to unwanted behaviour.

If, following medication changes and evaluation by a specialist, a child is still felt to be experiencing significant learning or behavioural difficulties, then it is possible to have what is called a 'statement' made of a child's needs. This can be initiated by a parent or a teacher, but preferably a joint decision to undertake this procedure should be made. Having a statement made involves gathering information about the child from the doctor, from the child's teacher and from the parents. In addition, a child may undergo a psychological assessment. This may involve him or her being given special tests to explore abilities such as language and memory. The tests, given by psychologists, are used to help them judge whether they think a child's achievements at school are in keeping with his or her overall ability and his or her age. Results from these tests may enable reasonable expectations about academic goals to be made. A written document will be compiled, and this is called the statement. In it, recommendations will be made about a child's needs and about appropriate educational input. The local education authority is then legally bound to make special educational provision for a child if this is considered necessary. This is likely to take place within the school which the child attends, and only very rarely will a recommendation be made for placement elsewhere. Indeed, it is government policy to educate the majority of children within mainstream education, and placements at special schools are today relatively infrequently made.

Special schooling is more likely to take place if factors additional to epilepsy exist, such as severe physical or mental handicap. There are three special schools catering for children with epilepsy in the United Kingdom, and one special assessment centre. The latter offers short-term schooling while a child undergoes assessment of their epilepsy, perhaps over a period of a few weeks or a few months. The other three schools can provide more long-term education, but they generally cater for children who have multiple handicaps in addition to their epilepsy.

Towards the end of a child's school career he or she will be entered for examinations, such as the GCSE. This can be a stressful time for all children, but it can also be an excellent learning experience. Undertaking examinations helps children face difficulties and attempt to overcome them. A diagnosis of epilepsy should not be a reason for missing examinations. It is possible that fit frequency may increase with the stress due to exams, but avoidance of stressful events, once begun, will result in a fairly restricted lifestyle.

YOUNG ADULTHOOD

The age of sixteen can be considered a crossroad. Do young people stay on at school or do they go to work? If a person with epilepsy has been academically successful, as many are, and has obtained good examination passes, then consideration of undertaking 'A' levels should be made. A diagnosis of epilepsy should not prevent anyone considering going to college or university if he or she has the required grades at 'A' level. Many young people with epilepsy do go to university and obtain degrees and higher degrees. The available evidence, although limited, suggests a positive attitude towards epilepsy at colleges and universities.

Openness is best, and discussions with the medical officer based at the college may be valuable. This can result in lower floor accommodation near to the medical centre if this is felt to be needed. Surveys suggest, however, that young people with epilepsy are reluctant to reveal their diagnosis, and ultimately this must be their decision. Certain academic courses are more difficult to get on to with a history of epilepsy. Young people with epilepsy may find it difficult to enrol for science degrees and those involving physical education. Selection of an appropriate university course is something that should be undertaken with care, and should be considered well in advance of completion of studies at school. Most schools have a careers adviser, or access to a careers adviser, who can help an individual make appropriate decisions.

Going to university can be the first experience of living away from home. A sensible life-style is to be recommended. People with epilepsy should try to avoid loss of sleep which may arise if revision for examinations is left until the last minute. Too much alcohol when completion of examinations is celebrated should also be avoided.

Further education is not solely confined to universities and polytechnics. There is a variety of courses available generally at colleges of further education and technical colleges. These include courses for individuals with learning difficulties. The person with epilepsy may have missed out at school due to fits, resulting in significant time away from classes. Local colleges may run more practically orientated courses where individuals find they have a particular skill. A careers officer at school will be able to advise on the availability and suitability of courses.

Going to Work

Having a job is more than a means of earning money. Our work can provide us with a sense of identity, and indeed it is often the second piece of information we provide to somebody we have just met. Work also gives us a sense of purpose and a sense of being needed. Finding appropriate work to meet our individual skills and talents can be very important, and can influence our enjoyment of and satisfaction with life. Research on epilepsy suggests a low rate of accidents due to epileptic fits, and attendance and performance records for people with epilepsy are higher than average. It would be wrong, however, to give the impression that no problems exist. Some people with epilepsy do experience difficulties in obtaining suitable employment, particularly at times of high unemployment. Epilepsy does reduce career options, and a problem experienced by some individuals is under-use of their skills.

It is very difficult to generalise about which job should or should not be undertaken, since this is a very individual thing. Each person with epilepsy must seriously consider the nature of his or her own attacks and make a realistic decision about their likely impact on employment choices. It is important that people consider how their fits are at the time they are applying for jobs, and not how they would hope their fit control might be following drug changes.

There are some occupations which will be prohibited even if an individual has been free from seizures without medication for many years. Certain careers are not possible where there has ever been a history of epilepsy, and these include being an airline pilot, joining the Royal Navy, being a professional diver, and working in the fire service in an active capacity. In addition, a person with epilepsy would not be permitted to work as a train driver or be involved in the maintenance of the tracks on the London underground. There are further jobs which would not be permitted if a fit has occurred after the age of 5 years. The majority of these jobs involve some form of professional driving, for example driving an ambulance, a heavy goods vehicle, or public service vehicles such as buses and taxis. A person with epilepsy would not be able to join the merchant navy and would probably experience difficulty in signing up for the army. Such barriers may seem unjust; however, they currently stand, and are unlikely to change substantially in the near future. If seizures are very well controlled or if attacks occur only at night career options are increased. For instance, training to become a nurse becomes a possibility, although certain branches such as midwifery or working in intensive care units may not be possible as ultimate career goals. People with well-controlled epilepsy can train to become teachers. However, even then some restrictions will be encountered, and undertaking physical education, cookery and science subjects which can involve the handling of potentially dangerous chemical substances will probably not be permitted. Epilepsy is not a bar to becoming a doctor, although again it may be unwise to pursue certain fields.

In general, the better controlled seizures are, the wider a person's employment chances. This is certainly the case for many semi- and unskilled jobs. Even if a person has experienced one seizure in the past three years, working as a window cleaner, or work involving scaffolding or unguarded machinery would be inappropriate choices as they might place the person with epilepsy at risk and also put other people in danger. In the same way, jobs which involve working in isolation at distant locations with poor communications may also be considered risky, depending on the nature and type of attack experienced. For some individuals, regular sleep contributes to good seizure control, and this may become disrupted, for example, by doing shift work. This may result in a shortage of sleep and fatigue, temporarily resulting in an increase in attacks. It may be particularly disruptive if an individual experiences only night-time seizures. For such individuals, doing shift work may increase the likelihood of having an attack during the day as a result of their 'nodding off' due to tiredness.

It is not only the frequency of seizures that will need to be considered when selecting a job. The type of attack is also important. Individuals may be at an advantage if they have some form of warning which allows them to put down what they are doing and retire to a safe place. The duration of attacks will also need to be considered. If seizures are relatively short-lived, this may well influence selection of a job. If recovery is slow and there is any period of confusion, or if complex partial seizures are experienced involving a period of wandering or strange behaviour, then these factors may increase the risk associated with the attack for the person with epilepsy, and indeed their work colleagues. Careful consideration must be given to career choices and individuals must be realistic about the impact their epilepsy may have on the jobs they are considering.

In the last ten to twenty years there has been a significant increase in the number of jobs available involving new technology; working with computers, word processors and so on. Indeed, in many ways these jobs seem very suitable for people with epilepsy and should be seriously considered when making career choices. Unfortunately, a misconception seems to have arisen that working with a computer monitor could place people at risk and could result in an increase in seizures. This is not the case, and only a small percentage of people who have photosensitive epilepsy will be expected to have seizures triggered by working on a computer. It is possible for those individuals with such epilepsy to have this established long before they make their career choices. Indeed, the new technology offers increased opportunities for those with epilepsy to work in safe environments and realise their potential.

There is a small group of people with epilepsy who experience frequent seizures or severe attacks, in which self-injury is a problem. If individuals fall into this group, obtaining suitable employment may be difficult, particularly if they are without academic or vocational qualifications. Individuals falling into this category who are experiencing great difficulty obtaining work may find that the local job centre recommends they pay a visit to a disablement resettlement officer (DRO). These are people employed by the Manpower Services Commission, which is a branch of the Department of Employment dealing with the recruitment, training and special services which facilitate the return to work of the unemployed.

The DRO's role is to try to find placements for adults with disabilities. They can be very helpful in outlining work possibilities that may be available. DROs may recommend an individual attends an employment rehabilitation centre for a short period, usually a maximum of a few months. Such centres evaluate work skills, and include the opportunity to try different types of work including clerical, electronic and more practical skills. The range of work offered varies slightly from centre to centre. Currently there are twenty-seven such centres in the United Kingdom. It is the experience of the authors that DROs and employment rehabilitation centres vary enormously in their understanding of epilepsy. Individuals who attend such centres should have a clear understanding of their own epilepsy so that they can present it to others and help dispel any misconceptions which they may have. Some people may also want to contact the Employment Medical Advisory Service, which employs specially trained doctors and nursing staff who can be approached to discuss the medical advisability of certain jobs. The location of an individual's nearest regional advisor can be obtained from a DRO.

Following assessment, a recommendation may be made that an individual register as disabled. There exists in the United Kingdom a quota scheme whereby employers who have more than twenty people working for them are obliged to have 3 per cent of their work force made up of people who are registered as disabled. It may be difficult for a person with epilepsy to decide whether they want to become registered as disabled, and some people are very loath to do this. Unfortunately, failure to register as disabled will bar individuals from eligibility for the quota scheme. If seizures are particularly handicapping, the DRO may recommend a sheltered work environment. In the past, the trend was sheltered workshops where groups of disabled people would work together in the same environment. Remploy is an organisation which runs factories for workers with disabilities. Local authorities and voluntary organisations also run sheltered workshops. In more recent years there seems to have been a move away from sheltered placements towards trying to obtain work for those with a disability in normal work environments. Job Introduction and Job Rehearsal schemes are two placement programmes which involve working in more normal environments. Details of existing schemes and their availability in any locality can be obtained from a DRO.

There are many factors apart from seizure frequency that can influence whether an individual is successful in obtaining employment, and it is important for people with epilepsy to bear these in mind when they look for work. A person's qualifications, both academic and past work experience, will also be important. It is vital that a career has been selected which is realistic in terms of an individual's aptitude and educational background.

Most jobs involve going for an interview, and coping with this situation demands fairly well-developed social skills in order to make the right impression. These skills can be learned and practised, and in addition it is an asset if an individual has a good understanding of his or her epilepsy so that a good explanation can be given to the prospective employer. In particular, people must feel confident about correcting any misinformation the employer may have. Practising interviews with friends, families and in front of a mirror may be helpful. Tape-recording responses may also prove useful. If a person feels he is suitable for a particular job, he must try to convince the interviewer that his seizures will not interfere with his performance. It may help if the individual has a back-up letter from his doctor about the control of his seizures.

The way individuals feel about themselves (their self-image), is also important. If people have realistic ambitions and feel good about themselves, this can greatly influence the way they present themselves, and also have an effect on whether they obtain and hold down a job. Individuals should be aware of their own strengths so that they can convey these to the prospective employer. People should not expect employers to have negative views about epilepsy. Indeed, the majority of employers should be expected to be ignorant about the disorder. If people expect negative reactions to their epilepsy, this may result in them behaving in an aggressive or even hostile way during the interview, and this would soon be picked up by the interviewer.

We do not want to give the impression that prejudice against epilepsy is not a problem in the work market. It can occur, and individuals must be prepared to cope with disappointments, including frequent job rejections. On many occasions this may be due to strong competition for a job and may not be due to epilepsy. People with epilepsy must try to overcome disappointments when they occur and not let them result in despondency, as this can lead to apathy and hostility which will become only too apparent at the next interview.

A dilemma experienced by some people with epilepsy when applying for jobs is whether to declare their condition or not. Most jobs require the completion of an application document and this may include specific questions about health matters, and may even ask about epilepsy. Some people choose not to mention their condition but feel they may be better understood if they discuss it at the interview stage. In certain organisations and for certain jobs there is a move towards having information about health kept separate from other factors. Information about health would only be considered if an individual was thought to be suitable in all other respects for the job, and then only if it was felt relevant to the job. Unfortunately this is not common practice, although it is to be commended.

It is difficult to give general advice on declaration of epilepsy. If the form asks direct questions about epilepsy, some individuals feel a positive response might reduce their chances of being selected for the interview. In fact in certain instances it often seems appropriate not to disclose on the form but to wait for an interview to bring this up. In the interview situation an individual can discuss his epilepsy more fully, perhaps towards the end of the interview. At this time he can present an informed account of the nature of his attacks and make a strong argument that they would not interfere with the job. It is also hoped that by this time in the interview the individual would have already made a favourable impression upon the interview panel.

If a person is offered a job and has not revealed his epilepsy, there may be unfortunate consequences including justifiable dismissal. It may be extremely unlikely that fits will occur at work, but fear of being found out can increase stress and reduce work efficiency. If an employer knows about a person's epilepsy and what may happen (for example, that it will be a short-lived episode with prompt resumption of work duties), this will greatly ease the situation.

Whether an individual discusses his epilepsy with his or her work mates may be a more difficult decision and there are no hard and fast rules. It may be more appropriate to wait until he has been in the job for a while and feels comfortable with the people with whom he is working. Most people are usually very willing to help and to make allowances if they are told something about epilepsy. Work mates may be more sympathetic if they are aware of what happens in an attack and what is the appropriate course of action. Discussions with the personnel department or occupational health service may give helpful advice on the problem of disclosure. If a person has a fit at work and has concealed his epilepsy from his employer instant dismissal may result, and the person is legally in a very weak position.

If a person has his first fit at work, or at home during the period of employment, openness with the employer seems essential. It may be that the occupation is one in which having epilepsy places him at risk, and this is something that would need to be discussed with the employer, who should really attempt to find an alternative position to reduce the risk to both the person with epilepsy and the other employees. If a person has been in a job for more than two years, has a fit, and subsequently is dismissed, he or she is in a very strong position to claim for unfair dismissal.

Some employers fear that people with epilepsy are not eligible for pension schemes. These fears are unfounded, and most schemes in existence are capable of covering people with epilepsy. Indeed, it is stated by the Occupational Pensions Board that disabled people should have the same access to pension schemes as able-bodied people. Similarly, provided that an individual has selected his work carefully, he should also be covered by the insurance policy of his employer. Insurance companies in general have undertaken to include all disabled people, and this includes people with epilepsy, in the employer's liability insurance policy. When suitable employment for people with epilepsy has been selected there is no evidence that they are at risk of more accidents than other employees, and indeed, existing evidence suggests that they may experience fewer accidents. Individuals experiencing problems concerning pension schemes or insurance could contact their DRO. National voluntary organisations may also provide advice and support on these issues (*see* Useful Addresses, page 94).

Individuals with epilepsy naturally worry that taking drugs may influence their working capacity. Most available drugs, if taken regularly, should have minimal side-effects. People with epilepsy are in the best position to monitor their efficiency at work. If they feel that their concentration is not as good as it used to be, or they feel more tired or forgetful, then it might be appropriate for them to seek a review of their epilepsy. Similarly, if they begin to experience attacks in increasing frequency and they are taking tablets regularly, evaluation of their fits may be deemed appropriate.

Underemployment can occur in epilepsy. By this we mean that a person is in a post which is not sufficiently demanding of his experience or academic background. This may be because he or his employer feels that responsibility or other demands could bring on fits. This is unlikely, and paradoxically, responsibility can have a positive effect on fits and, of equal importance, on self-esteem. Sometimes the nature of an individual's attack results in his undertaking a less demanding job, and there may be no alternative to this. In this instance, although the job may be unrewarding, the person with epilepsy may be able to pursue more rewarding activities outside work hours.

Unemployment

Being out of work can be a difficult adjustment for anyone to make. Having a job helps us to structure our time. With no job, there is no

59

need to get up early, and people can easily slip into the habit of rising late and staying up into the early hours of the morning. Inactivity during the day can result in reduced motivation. Unemployment is easier to cope with if individuals can institute a regular life-style and find something constructive to do with their spare time. Participation in voluntary work and involvement with self-help groups for epilepsy or indeed for other disabilities can be rewarding. Some people with epilepsy experience an increase in fits if they are unemployed for a long time, and often this is due to boredom and inactivity.

People who are unemployed or in a lower income job may be entitled to some financial assistance. Major changes were made to social security benefits in April 1988. The following are some of the existing benefits to which people with epilepsy or their families may be eligible:

Invalidity benefit   Invalidity care allowance
Severe disablement allowance   Income support
Mobility allowance   Social fund
Attendance allowance

Entitlement will vary depending on past work record, current income and available savings. For further information on eligibility for these benefits an appointment should be made at the local social security office, or the Citizens' Advice Bureau may be contacted.

Friendships

Developing and maintaining friendships is an important human activity, and indeed we spend much of our lives engaged in social interactions of some sort. Having friends is something that may be taken for granted, but is soon appreciated when we receive support through difficult times in our lives. During adolescence and young adulthood the formation of friendships and the involvement in activities outside the family increases in frequency. Indeed, this is important for the development of self-identity and building of self-confidence. It is through this process that many individuals ultimately form intimate relationships. These relationships in turn provide the motivation to leave the parental home and to form families of our own. Epilepsy should not be allowed to disrupt this process, although at times individuals may encounter obstacles, some of which may seem more difficult to overcome than others.

The skills necessary to mix socially begin to develop in early childhood, particularly in our school years. If people experience fits during this time, later development may still not be a problem, provided that the child was not treated differently by parents, school teachers or school friends, and was allowed to take part in a wide range of activities. People experiencing difficulty during these years, for example by being teased, may become less confident in social situations. Parents may have been anxious about letting their children take part in a wide range of activities and this can result in a lack of experience in social settings.

Parental supervision continues at least into early adolescence, and it is helpful if individuals with epilepsy are not unduly restricted during this time. For all parents, adolescence can be a difficult developmental stage because it is traditionally a time when children break away and become more independent of the family. However, this is a necessary process, and should not be prevented because of epilepsy. If fits are not completely controlled, going out socially may involve some risk-taking. However, if a person's friends are aware of the seizures and know how to react to them, they will be just as capable of coping as the parents have been in the past.

Parents are not the only people to restrict a child's activities. Some young people experience embarrassment or fear about the possibility of having a fit in public. This is not an uncommon feeling, even when fits are well controlled. Such feelings can make individuals withdraw socially. It is important for psychological health and a person's enjoyment of life that he or she should try to overcome such feelings when they occur. If young people can be open with their friends, they will be more comfortable about being with others. By mixing with friends in a normal way, people with epilepsy can also do a great deal to improve public attitude, by showing that having epilepsy does not make a person an oddity.

Epilepsy should not prevent young people from undertaking the majority of leisure activities. This is particularly the case when the activities involve being with other people. Contrary to common belief, many individuals with epilepsy find that they are less likely to have seizures when they are engaged in recreational pursuits.

Another common misunderstanding of parents and young people with epilepsy is that flashing lights at discotheques and nightclubs will trigger fits. This is the case only for a minority of individuals who have a specific type of epilepsy, namely photosensitive epilepsy. Investigations can be undertaken to find out whether a person falls into this category. Even people with photosensitive epilepsy may not be at risk at the discotheque, since to cause a seizure, the lights need to flash faster than is usually the speed of most stroboscopes used at discotheques. In addition, it may be possible to reduce the fit-inducing properties of a flashing light by shutting one eye.

Social life may also revolve around a local pub or wine bar, and sooner or later concern may be raised about drinking alcohol. There is an interaction between alcohol and anticonvulsant medication, but this should not cause a problem if people drink in moderation. Indeed, drinking should always be undertaken in moderation, irrespective of a diagnosis of epilepsy. It is not only large quantities of alcohol which can induce fits, but also large amounts of liquids. People with epilepsy should be careful never to over-indulge as a result of pressure from others. An increase in fits is not likely to occur at the time of drinking, but rather on the following day. Heavy drinking can also be associated with an increase in fits due to a loss of sleep and missed tablets.

Epilepsy and Driving

Whether or not they will be able to drive is a major concern of young people with epilepsy. This is not surprising. Learning to drive and owning a car or borrowing a parent's car can be an important status symbol, a means of decreasing dependence on the family, and also a practical way of getting from A to B. This may be particularly valuable for those who live in remote areas where there is no regular transport. People with epilepsy are able to drive only if they have been fit-free for at least two years, or if they have had fits only during sleep for a period of three years. If individuals satisfy these criteria, there is an additional proviso that driving a vehicle is not likely to be a source of danger to the public.

If an individual fulfils these criteria, the first stage to obtaining a licence is to complete an application form, which can be obtained from a local post office. A further form will be sent requesting more information about seizures, and at this stage the person's doctor will also be asked to provide information. The person will be issued with a licence and will then be able to drive. It is possible that in the first instance the licence may be given for a defined period of time, such as one, two or maybe three years, after which the situation will be reviewed. If seizures are sufficiently well controlled for an individual to be able to drive, then avoidance of activities that may increase the likelihood of seizures is recommended. Long journeys should be avoided. Driving should not be undertaken if a person has had inadequate sleep. All alcohol should be avoided when driving.

If a person experiences a fit, he or she must stop driving immediately and notify the Driver and Motor Vehicle Licensing Centre (DVLC) in Swansea. It is the person's responsibility, and not that of the doctor, to do this. People must be very honest with themselves and not deny that a seizure has occurred. Anyone who continues to drive will not only be putting his own life at risk but potentially the lives of other motorists and pedestrians. People who continue to drive after seizures have occurred can be prosecuted. The length of the seizure does not matter, and even a short absence or an aura is sufficient to make driving illegal.

Some people will never have adequate seizure control to allow them to drive. Each time they seem to be near qualifying, for example being seizure-free for twenty-three months, they may experience another attack. This can be one of the biggest disappointments encountered by young people with epilepsy, and may be difficult to come to terms with. However, if individuals are developing their skills and forming friendships, there will be other people who can give them lifts to social events.

Sexual Development

Adolescence is not only a time of social development; it is also a time of sexual development. There is no evidence to suggest that having epilepsy significantly interferes with puberty in either sex. The onset of menstruation may be associated with an increase in seizures in some individuals. This may be due to hormonal changes, but bodily changes can also cause anxiety which may underlie an increase in seizures. If fits are observed to occur at the time of menstruation, this should be discussed with the doctor as it may have implications for treatment.

There is no reason why having epilepsy should prevent a person forming intimate relationships and having sexual intercourse. Reports of reduced sex drive and impotence accompanying epilepsy have been made, but there is limited research evidence to support this. Often, studies have been undertaken on rather unrepresentative groups of people with epilepsy, and it is unclear whether epilepsy is the underlying cause or there are other more potentially reversible causes. For example, a restricted upbringing and lack of sexual knowledge may cause problems. A fear of having a fit during intercourse is another concern which people may have. It is exceedingly unlikely that a seizure will occur at this time; however, if an individual's anxiety is aroused by such a fear, this will undoubtedly interfere with sexual performance. Anxiety is also likely to be increased if a person has not told his or her partner about the epilepsy. We would hope, however, that individuals embarking on a sexual relationship will have formed a close friendship where concerns such as these have been discussed openly.

Sexual difficulties can of course occur in people with epilepsy, just as they occur in people who do not have epilepsy. When problems arise, openness is of paramount importance. If one partner is experiencing problems and does not disclose them the situation is only made worse. Frank discussion can often help resolve or alleviate any difficulties. A problem involving sexual intercourse is a joint problem. If problems persist following open discussion, the couple should seek advice, and not just accept the difficulties as part and parcel of having epilepsy. The GP should be the first point of contact for such a problem.

Contraception is an important consideration for all couples who plan to have a sexually fulfilling relationship. A wide range of methods is currently available, the contraceptive pill having the widest popularity. There is no evidence to suggest that taking the pill adversely affects epilepsy. Anticonvulsant drugs, however, can influence the metabolism of the pill and reduce its effectiveness, thereby increasing the likelihood of pregnancy. Ineffective cover is most likely to happen with lower dose pills. The different forms of contraception should be discussed with the GP or the doctor at the local family planning clinic. Women on the pill who experience breakthrough bleeding should take this as an indication of the decreased reliability of this measure. Additional methods of contraception should be employed, and the matter raised at their next appointment with the family planning services or with the GP.

ADULTHOOD

Starting a Family

Deciding whether and when to have children warrants careful consideration by all couples. Starting a family brings changes in life-style, such as increased responsibility, and often decreased income. The psychological and practical implications of having children need to be discussed. Uncertainties may be increased if either partner has epilepsy, and worries should not be bottled up. If there are any concerns about having children, they should be talked through and a joint decision made.

A question of major concern to couples must be, 'Will our child have fits?' There is no easy answer, but evidence suggests that heredity plays only a minor role, and most children born to mothers or fathers with epilepsy do not develop seizures. There are some circumstances where there is an increased risk of the child inheriting a tendency to develop fits, and this occurs when a low seizure threshold is inherited. Whether this applies or not will depend on the nature of the parent's epilepsy. Before starting a family it is recommended that couples discuss this with their GP, who may if necessary refer them for special genetic counselling. If both parents have a history of epilepsy, the chances that the child will develop seizures are greater. It must also be remembered that if both parents have seizures which are not well controlled, there may be practical implications for the care of their children.

Once potential parents have decided to start a family, have talked it over and feel satisfied that they have received sufficient advice about inheritance, they often still have worries that having epilepsy may decrease fertility. There is no evidence to suggest that having seizures affects the production of eggs or causes hormonal problems that can influence fertility. Concerns may also be raised that the pregnancy may be difficult. Women with epilepsy usually have uncomplicated pregnancies with normal deliveries and healthy children. Antenatal classes are to be recommended, and may prove very beneficial, particularly those including sessions on relaxation.

Will taking drugs affect the developing baby? There is increased awareness that the developing foetus is most vulnerable in the early weeks after conception, particularly the first three months. During this time, smoking, intake of alcohol, inadequate diet and exposure to infectious diseases can place the developing child at risk. It is thought that some anticonvulsants may increase the risk of babies developing abnormalities, although the research findings are not very clear cut. It is therefore advisable for a visit to be made to the GP or specialist before conception so that medication can be reviewed in the light of the decision to become pregnant. This forward planning allows sufficient time for drug changes to be made if this is felt appropriate. Medication should never be reduced without seeking advice, as this is potentially dangerous. Seizures during pregnancy can be damaging and have been associated with birth abnormalities.

Most anticonvulsants are used up more quickly during pregnancy. This means that the level of the drug can fall, which may increase the likelihood of seizures. This is another reason why it is important to seek medical advice before conception. Not only can drug changes be made if necessary, but the doctor can begin to monitor the level of the drugs in the body and make sure that any significant drop in drug level can be offset against increased medication. Similarly, following the birth, blood levels again need checking, since an increase in medication during pregnancy can result in the mother becoming intoxicated after the birth. Some women, irrespective of changes in medication, experience a change in seizure control. This is not consistent, but a significant proportion experience improved control during pregnancy. It is not clear why this happens.

The Baby

Traces of anticonvulsant drugs do appear in the breast milk. However, the concentrations are very low, and it is important to remember that the baby will already have been exposed to them before birth. Breast-feeding is therefore generally safe. If seizures are not well controlled, bottle feeding provides mothers with an alternative. One advantage of bottle feeding is that both parents can share in the feeding of the child, and this can have practical and some psychological advantages.

It is unlikely that having fits will interfere greatly with an individual's ability to look after a young child, provided the attacks are well controlled. If fits are less well controlled, risks do exist. The nature of these risks depends on the type of attacks which an individual experiences, when they occur, and which parent has them. If the parent feeding the child has uncontrolled seizures, we recommend that feeding is undertaken while sitting on the floor with the back to the wall and adequate support.

A new baby in a family can mean a time of broken sleep. Loss of sleep can lead to an increase in seizures for some people with epilepsy. It is therefore very important that if a parent with epilepsy experiences significant sleep loss an attempt is made to compensate for this during the day.

If seizures are not completely controlled, the other partner may be able to undertake certain activities with the baby or, better still, these activities (for example, bathing, changing nappies and feeding) can be undertaken together. Joint parental ventures such as these can contribute to the psychological development of a child and greatly increase the enjoyment of parenthood. If activities such as bathing have to be undertaken by one parent alone, risks can be minimised by using very little water and giving the baby a sponge bath. Similarly, changing nappies can be undertaken on the floor rather than on a table. Other safety measures exist which are important for all parents. These include fire-guards, play-pens, stair gates, and cooker-guards. Some people have adapted prams so that if the person pushing them has a fit, the pram will automatically stop. However, the authors are not aware of a commercially available device which will do this.

Health visitors may have useful practical suggestions about ways of adapting a home to increase the safety of the child. Parents must be careful to keep their pills well out of the reach of young children, and particularly in the early years, should try to avoid the child watching while they take them. Young children love to copy the behaviour of their parents, and indeed this is very important for their development. When the child is older, the reason for taking the tablets can be explained.

Should children of parents with epilepsy have the recommended inoculations? Doctors usually advise that all inoculations with the exception of the whooping cough vaccine are safe. In the case of inoculation for whooping cough, expert advice may be needed and this can be discussed with the GP.

As children get older, concern may arise as to how they will cope when a parent has a seizure. There is no easy answer to this question; however, in most written accounts by parents with epilepsy, it seems to be the case that even from a very early age children can cope very well in this situation. Children can readily be taught the appropriate steps to take, for example not to panic, and to stand close by.

Household Safety

Most accidents occur within the home and garden. Often they result from careless errors or oversights. We give here some suggestions about reducing the likelihood of accidents within the home, which apply as much to people without epilepsy as to those with epilepsy. Common sense will reduce the risk of injury.

Let us begin in the kitchen. If seizures are frequent, the ideal solution to reduce the risk of burns when cooking is to use a microwave oven. A wide range of models is available, and also a large number of recipes, including many exotic foreign and elaborate meals which can be cooked entirely in a microwave. They are not as restrictive as some people imagine. Gas cookers have advantages and disadvantages – they can, for example, be easily turned off, but the naked flame can result in burns, particularly if contact is made with clothing during a fall. Electric cookers have no naked flame but they do take longer to cool down when switched off and this too can result in burns. An eye-level grill may be a problem as these can be easily tipped over. When cooking, it is safer to use the back burners with handles of saucepans pointing backwards, never sticking out where they may be accidentally knocked, causing spillage of food and accidents. When serving food it is safer to bring plates to the stove rather than lift a pan of hot food to the plate.

The need to eat healthy food is increasingly being impressed upon us. However, from time to time it is not harmful to have fried foods, and chips should not be prohibited. People who have a passion for such food should consider investing in a good electric deep fat fryer. This places them at less risk than would a chip pan on the cooker. Other electrical gadgets such as electric toasters and coffee makers can also increase safety in the home.

If seizures are not completely controlled, the possibility of drowning in the bath is a hazard which must be recognised. Shallow baths are advised and if the risk of a seizure exists, people with epilepsy should let somebody know when they are taking a bath. Ideally, a shower unit improves safety, particularly if carefully planned. The bathroom can be one of the smallest rooms in the house, particularly if there is a separate toilet. For this reason it is sometimes an advantage for people to have doors which open outwards. This can reduce problems in the event of someone having an attack and falling against the door. We would also recommend that in order to improve access in the case of an attack people with epilepsy should not lock themselves into the bathroom or toilet. An 'engaged' notice on the door could be used to prevent the entry of any unwanted intruders.

The risk of falling out of bed is probably not very great, but it can be minimised by having low-level divans. Futons (mattresses on the floor) are becoming fashionable and they can be particularly useful where space is limited. If individuals do not wish to have a low bed, an extra-wide bed can reduce the risk of falling out. Where there is a real risk that this will happen it is advisable to have soft carpet or mats fitted round the bed. For individuals who suffer nocturnal seizures it may be sensible to invest in safety pillows which reduce the risk of suffocation, but for the majority of people with epilepsy such precautions should not be necessary.

The risk from open fires can be reduced by using fire-guards. These are certainly to be recommended for people who have young children. Central heating is, however, probably one of the safest ways of heating a home, particularly if radiators are reasonably flush against the wall. Fixed lighting is also to be recommended. Wall lights cannot be knocked over and also result in more space in rooms. Foam sofas are to be avoided (this applies generally) particularly if the person with epilepsy smokes. A fit occurring whilst the person is smoking could result in a fire. Carpets should be soft and easy to clean. Trailing flexes should be avoided in order to prevent people tripping over them. If seizures are uncontrollable, windows and doors fitted with toughened glass can be worthwhile.

Some safety precautions may be needed outside the home. If full seizure control has not been achieved, the wearing of a 'Medic Alert' bracelet or necklace may be advisable. 'Medic Alert' is a charitable organisation which was founded almost forty years ago. There is a once-in-a-lifetime membership fee (£5.95 in 1988). A small additional cost may be charged for updating details, for example changing one's address. The cost covers a specially engraved bracelet or necklace which contains details of the person's medical problem and also a telephone number. People coming to the assistance of someone having a fit outside the home are then in a position to phone the number and obtain more information. The address of this organisation is given in Useful Addresses (page 95). It has to be acknowledged that the general public do not always notice 'Medic Alert' and similar tags. Even if noticed, people do not always know how to react. Nationwide publicity might improve this situation.

Leisure Time

Whether people with epilepsy marry and have a family, or remain single, they will certainly wish to take holidays from time to time. Epilepsy should not be a bar to taking trips away from home, but certain precautions may be advisable. It is most important for people to ensure that they have sufficient medication for the duration of their holidays. Epilepsy is no bar to going abroad and most countries have no regulations concerning entry for holiday purposes, although this has not always been the case.

Air travel has not been associated with an increase in seizures: however, long trips may be associated with disrupted sleep patterns. If individuals do not make adjustments to compensate for loss of sleep, their seizure threshold may be reduced temporarily. Anyone travelling by air is advised to keep their entire supply of tablets in their hand luggage. Placing some medication in their main luggage results in a risk, albeit very small, that their baggage may not arrive as promptly at their destination or may even decide to arrive at an alternative venue! For people travelling alone, it may be advisable to inform the airline of their epilepsy if there is a likelihood of having a seizure. Some airlines may request information from a doctor about the nature of a person's epilepsy.

It is advisable for people with epilepsy to take a letter with them on holiday, giving details of their seizures and medication. Where appropriate translations may be required when visits are made to non-English speaking countries. This should help people's passage through customs and avoid misunderstandings about carrying medication. In some countries there are subtle differences in drug names, and this can cause considerable problems if an individual is unfortunate enough to lose his tablets or decides to stay for a longer period. It is therefore advisable before going on holiday to try to find out what the medication names are in the country being visited. For example, in South America Epilem is the commercial name for phenytoin while in this country Epilim is the trade name for sodium valproate.

People travelling abroad to EEC countries should be able to reclaim any medical expenses incurred by completing a form E111 before they go. However, even in the EEC it is probably advisable to have additional insurance cover. Having epilepsy should not prevent a person obtaining an adequate holiday insurance policy. Anyone experiencing difficulties should shop around: the British Epilepsy Association has details of insurance companies offering travel insurance to people with epilepsy (*see* Useful Addresses).

Some people, particularly those with their own home, may decide that holiday time is best spent looking after their property. For people with epilepsy who are unemployed time may be used profitably in carrying out 'do-it-yourself' repairs on the house. People with epilepsy must be realistic as to which activities are appropriate to be undertaken, given the nature of their fits. Working on high ladders replacing roof tiles is not advisable in any event, nor is working with a chainsaw (although this probably applies also to a lot of people without epilepsy). Gardening would seem a relatively safe occupation, but some precautions may be necessary. Special power-breakers can reduce risks if people are using electric lawnmowers.

For some people, leisure activities include sports. Indeed, we are becoming an increasingly health-conscious society. Eating well and being physically fit and active is as good for people with epilepsy as for everybody else. There is no evidence to suggest that exercise necessarily makes seizures worse. The recommendations regarding sporting activities at school discussed on page 47 should be noted.

LATER LIFE

Most of the areas covered so far apply to people of all ages. People with long-standing epilepsy will already have made adjustments so that their seizures have a minimal influence on their lives. It may, however, be very hard to adapt when seizures occur for the first time later in life. People will already be established in their life-style and their line of work. A diagnosis of epilepsy may have significant implications for occupation and may prevent the person from driving. For those people who have been employed for many years with the same firm, the impact of seizures on their employment must be considered. It does not necessarily mean a change of job. If the attacks place the person at risk, alternative work within the firm should be found where possible. Individuals finding themselves out of work for the first time in their 50s may experience considerable difficulty obtaining work. It may be that people falling into this group have to make a career change or even accept some form of redundancy on health grounds, and adjust to life without work.

Later life is a time when, for those with a family, children are growing up and leaving home. This can be a stressful period, and this may influence attacks in some individuals. At a time when children are leaving home, a person's own parents may be becoming older and increasingly frail, and may need looking after. It is also a time when people may become grandparents. Epilepsy should not prevent individuals looking after grandchildren or caring for an elderly relative. If attacks are not well controlled and are unpredictable, then precautions should be taken, and carrying young children or being on one's own for long periods of time are probably not wise.

For women, the later years bring the menopause, when a series of biochemical and psychological changes occur, following which it is impossible to have children. This generally happens between the mid-40s and mid-50s. The commoner symptoms of these changes are hot flushes and night sweats; less commonly experienced are headaches, dizzy spells, and depression. Many women, however, do not experience any major prolonged distressing symptoms, and for those that do, hormone replacement therapy has proved to be very helpful. There is no evidence of notable association between epilepsy and menopausal changes, nor is there any evidence that hormone replacement therapy influences seizure control or metabolism of epileptic drugs, although this has not been the focus of much research.

For those individuals in employment, retirement is a hurdle to be faced in later years. With increasing life expectancy, many people live several decades following retirement. People often do not appreciate to what extent work provides them with a structured day. Adjusting to this loss of routine is something which does not necessarily come easily, and people can find themselves at a loss for something to do and may feel socially isolated. Planning for retirement is recommended, with or without epilepsy. Indeed, some firms and organisations have classes to prepare people for this.

It is important to remember that for some individuals, inactivity can be associated with an increase in seizure frequency. Loss of a daily routine may also make people less reliable in taking their medication. There is also some evidence that as the body grows older, the metabolism of anticonvulsant drugs may change, and for some individuals a decrease in medication is indicated. People with epilepsy must monitor their own condition, and if they feel that they are unduly drowsy or that their concentration is poor, this should be discussed with their doctor. Epilepsy is not a static condition, and changes in treatment may be required at different times in an individual's life. There is also evidence that as everyone gets older, memory tends to become somewhat less efficient. For this reason, people may need to rely on special techniques such as those discussed in the next chapter to avoid missing tablets. It is to be hoped that the later years for a person with epilepsy should be a time for enjoyment and activity. Epilepsy should be taking a back seat, and for those who have had a family there is time to enjoy the development of grandchildren and even great-grandchildren.

6
Psychological Problems

ANXIETY

Anxiety is a feeling we all experience from time to time. We become anxious when we are unsure of what will happen or when something is about to happen. Anxiety is an appropriate and healthy reaction. It prepares us for uncertainty and can result in improved concentration and performance, for example, anxiety before an examination, a job interview, or an important meeting. When anxiety levels get too high or anxious feelings persist for a long time, its beneficial effects are lost, and a person's ability to function and to cope can deteriorate rapidly. Sometimes, anxiety can become overwhelming and, seemingly out of the blue, a person may feel intense fear and an inability to react psychologically or physically. Such episodes are generally called 'panic attacks'. For most people, anxiety is less obvious but feelings of tiredness, restlessness, headaches and edginess may all be unwanted symptoms.

Epilepsy is a condition that is characterised by the suddenness and unpredictability of the seizure. It would be very useful if people could book in their fits to happen at a particular time, for example 7 p.m. on a Thursday evening before they go out. Unfortunately, people with epilepsy are never sure when or where a fit may occur. This feeling of uncertainty may exist even if they have not had a fit for years or even decades. Having epilepsy means that people have to learn to live with such unpredictability. Most people cope with the uncertainty of their fits and learn to overcome feelings of anxiety when these threaten to be overwhelming. Indeed, people may find that high levels of anxiety can trigger fits. People worry about having a fit, the worry triggers an attack, which in turn increases levels of anxiety about having another fit, and so a vicious circle can be formed. When anxiety levels are high, not only can they influence seizure control, but they will certainly affect the individual's ability to cope at work and in social situations.

It is possible to be anxious and not realise it. Physical signs of anxiety include heart pounding, sweating, butterflies in the stomach, headaches, shallow breathing, restlessness and difficulty sleeping. Individuals may feel frightened and panicky, and feel they are losing control. Negative thoughts occur, such as 'I can't cope', 'It's going to be awful', and 'I will make a fool of myself'. Such thoughts can contribute to feelings of anxiety, as can negative attitudes. An attitude refers to the beliefs individuals have about things. Attitudes develop gradually as we are growing up with our family and friends. People may not be aware they are holding fairly negative attitudes. Some people with epilepsy feel that they very much have to prove themselves to other people to show they are 'normal'. This can result in striving twice as hard as other people, and such an attitude can increase levels of anxiety.

People may find that they are avoiding social situations and staying at home because it makes them feel less anxious. If people with epilepsy are behaving in such a way, it is important to question whether it is because of anxiety. If it is, and if it is not tackled early, then a person's self-confidence will become eroded and self-esteem lowered. Depression may result.

There are certain times when we are particularly at risk of experiencing anxiety. Stressful life-events such as taking examinations, changing job, the death of a relative are examples of these. Indeed, events which may seem to be positive, such as getting married or going on holiday have all been associated with increased stress levels. Life-events are generally considered to be relatively short-lived but there are other experiences that can be more long-term in nature and in the effect they have upon our mood. Anxiety has been associated with long periods of unemployment, with relationship problems and with other instances such as financial difficulties and also chronic boredom. People with epilepsy must question whether there are events or strains in their lives that might be increasing their feelings of anxiety.

If a person is anxious, what can be done? An important step in reducing levels of anxiety is for the person to have a good understanding of his or her epilepsy and seizures, including what they actually do during an attack. Having such knowledge can greatly increase an individual's feelings of being in control. People with epilepsy should avoid concealing it from those with whom they are in regular contact. We have come across families where the existence of epilepsy is not even acknowledged between family members. People should feel at their most relaxed when they are with their family, and this will not be the case if they deny the existence of epilepsy. At work and in other social situations secrecy about fits can result in chronic anxiety, stemming from the fear of being 'found out'.

An important step towards coping with anxiety is to understand when it occurs and why it occurs, that it is a normal reaction which can get out of hand, and that it is something that people can learn to overcome. The most widespread technique for combating anxiety is learning to relax. Being able to relax is not something that everybody finds easy, and it is certainly not a skill that we are born with. Some people make the mistake of confusing relaxation with being inactive. It is possible to be fairly inactive while experiencing significant amounts of anxiety. It should be possible for people with epilepsy to teach themselves how to relax, and there is a wealth of reading material and audio-tapes which take the individual step-by-step through the process of relaxing. Some useful references for reading are given in the back of the book (page 93).

Negative thoughts that can result from anxiety also need to be worked upon. Individuals need to be aware of what they are thinking, to stop occasionally at different points in the day to question different thoughts going on in their heads. As we have mentioned, people sometimes find their head is full of statements such as 'It is going to be awful', 'I can't cope', 'I am going to fail'. Such thoughts are extremely unhelpful, and it is important to work on them and to replace them with more positive thoughts and attitudes. People must learn to tell themselves to be calm, that they will be able to cope with a particular situation, and that nothing awful is going to happen. This procedure, like relaxation, may seem awkward and artificial, but with time most people find that they need to work on negative attitudes less and less as more positive ones become prominent.

People must also be aware of their attitudes towards epilepsy and other people's reactions to epilepsy. Individuals must question whether their attitudes are realistic, or whether they are perhaps self-defeating. In particular, it is important to be aware of the way one feels at times of stressful life-events. Anxiety can be a normal reaction at such times, but people must be careful to keep it in check so that it does not have too great a detrimental effect on their coping skills. By learning to relax, people become more adept at spotting the early signs of anxiety, and they are then in a position to take steps to prevent such feelings becoming overwhelming and to prevent them interfering with their lives.

It is possible that anxiety has already become overwhelming, and the person with epilepsy may feel unable to try to overcome it on his or her own. People who experience such feelings may come to feel a prisoner in their own home. For these individuals support from others can be helpful. Epilepsy support and self-help groups have a useful function in this respect. By talking with other people who have epilepsy or experience of epilepsy, people will find that they are not the only one who feels this way. Such discussions can provide individuals with the resources to get back in control of things. To seek advice from a support group does not mean that an individual has to become a regular group member, although this is an option that people may like to pursue. Most groups are willing to provide support on a one-to-one basis which could even be done simply over the telephone. Useful addresses are given on pages 94–95.

When feelings of anxiety have really become entrenched, this will lead to other psychological problems. People may feel so incapacitated as to be unable to initiate contact with a self-help group. This is a time when they should visit their GP. He or she can evaluate the situation and the GP is in a position to refer people for professional intervention from the psychological or psychiatric services. Psychologists, psychiatrists, and other professionals are trained to help people suffering with various psychological problems. There is a wide range of psychotherapies that can be undertaken.

Drugs do exist which can reduce feelings of anxiety. Tranquillisers and sleeping pills are among the most commonly prescribed drugs today. These drugs may help people to cope during a particularly stressful time, for instance following the death of a spouse, but they can have disadvantages if taken for too long. They have been associated with side-effects such as fatigue, impaired concentration and memory problems. There is also increasing awareness that such drugs can become addictive, and it may be very difficult to stop taking them. Indeed, the side-effects of withdrawal can be more distressing than the feelings of anxiety for which the drugs were originally prescribed. In the first instance, we feel that psychological interventions such as those outlined above are to be preferred in epilepsy. People with epilepsy may already have to take a number of drugs. Furthermore, if individuals are able to overcome unwanted feelings of anxiety without recourse to drugs, this can result in a sense of achievement which can greatly boost self-esteem. It will also give people the confidence that they can overcome difficult periods on their own, and will better equip them to cope with inevitable future stresses.

DEPRESSION

We all experience feelings of sadness and disappointment during the course of our lives in the same way that we feel happy when things are going well. The term depression usually refers to feelings of unhappiness and feeling down that are quite severe and persistent, lasting several weeks or more. Often, depression can be associated with feelings of loss. A clear example is the grief felt when a close friend or relative dies. Other losses that may result in such feelings include divorce, being sacked or becoming unemployed. Individuals may feel that they have lost out unfairly because of their epilepsy. They may feel that their job is undemanding, or perhaps they are unemployed. Epilepsy may be limiting their independence because they need to rely on others for transport, or people may feel dependent because they have to rely on tablets to control their seizures. An epileptic fit is in itself a form of loss of control which may increase the individual's feelings of dependency on others. If a diagnosis of epilepsy is made during adult years, a number of losses can occur during a short space of time, and it may be difficult to cope with these. For example, people may change or lose their job, have to stop driving and experience financial difficulties. It may be difficult to accept and adjust to these.

Depression is something which can be manifest in various ways. People may find that they are tearful for apparently no reason at all. They may lose interest in things and find themselves withdrawing from friends and family. People may sit for hours doing nothing, and may even take to their beds for long periods of time. They may feel drained of energy or lose their appetite. There may be difficulty getting off to sleep, and early waking can be a problem. Sometimes people are quite unaware that they have become depressed, and it is often family and friends who are living with them who become concerned. When people get depressed they can be difficult to live with, and relatives and friends may lose patience when they find their entreaties to 'pull yourself together' do not have the desired effect.

Individual feelings may also reveal significant depression. People may feel worthless and inadequate, and come to despise themselves. Guilt is another common experience. People may find that they are brooding over things from the past, and they may come to blame themselves for events that have gone wrong. Some individuals may even see developing epilepsy as some form of punishment because of their worthlessness. People may come to feel responsible for events and distress caused to their family and attribute them all to the fact that they have epilepsy. Thoughts may go round in their head such as 'I should have done that', 'I should never have responded in that way', or 'I can never be forgiven for what I have done' and so on. Not only may people feel bad about the past, but they may have no positive feelings about the future. They may feel hopeless, such that they do not feel that anything they do or say can change their situation. Indecision can be another feeling that is experienced. This is often related to low self-esteem. People come not to trust themselves to make the right decision, and so do nothing.

Most people are able to overcome feelings of depression on their own or with the support of their family and friends. There is no reason why people with epilepsy should be any different in this respect. One thing people may find beneficial is to work on their inactivity. Being depressed can result in no desire to do anything. When inactivity reaches its peak people may not be taking care of themselves properly. They may not care what they look like and may not attend to important things such as personal hygiene. This sort of sequence needs to be broken and stopped. The following activities have been reported to be helpful in reducing feelings of depression:

- Talking to somebody
- Writing letters

- Going for a walk
- Helping somebody out
- Seeing a friend

We recommend that when depressed, people select one activity which is likely to prove easy to undertake. One form of action could be to contact a self-help group. This course of action was also suggested when we discussed anxiety. Attendance of such a group may result in the person finding that other people feel or have felt in the same way, and have been able to overcome it.

It is not only a person's actions that need to be worked upon, but more importantly perhaps in depression, a person's thoughts. People must learn ways of dealing with negative thoughts, because they can maintain low mood and depressed behaviour. Individuals may be unaware of the sorts of thoughts that occupy their mind. We recommend that people learn to listen to the way they are thinking. At first people should note down what they are thinking during the day. Monitoring thoughts, like learning to relax, is not something that comes easily to us, and we would urge people not to give up doing this too soon. When people begin to look at their thoughts they may well find many of them to be unjustified. People who are depressed have a tendency to over-generalise. For example, they may think that because an unpleasant thing has happened once, it will always happen to them. People may have gone for a job interview and been rejected. This may result in a thought such as, 'I will never get a job again because I have epilepsy', or worse still, 'I can't do anything because I have epilepsy'. Such thoughts are unwarranted, resulting in a person becoming more depressed.

Analysing thoughts may also reveal that individuals are over-personalising situations. Somebody may cancel a visit and the person may interpret this as being because they do not want to see them. Examining thoughts may also reveal that individuals are constantly searching for answers – 'Why has this happened?' People may feel that there must be an answer to everything, when in fact this may not be the case. Such individuals may spend hours, days or weeks going over something when in fact no single answer exists.

People who feel depressed must also question whether they are focusing too much on negative things. 'I didn't do that properly',

'I won't be able to do this', 'Nothing good ever happens to me'. With some effort, people who are depressed can eventually generate some positive thoughts. This may not come easily at first but with determination most people can come up with some positive qualities or positive experiences. People should aim to focus increasingly on these more positive aspects and avoid focusing on negative interpretations of things going on around them.

Coming to terms with epilepsy and the consequences of having epilepsy is not something that will happen overnight. Having epilepsy does not have to ruin a person's life, and many people learn to adjust to the disorder and to see it as an inconvenience that has to be lived with. Where all attempts to overcome feelings of worthlessness fail, we suggest a visit to a GP. He or she is concerned about the mental well-being as well as the physical well-being of people. If the GP feels the situation warrants more specialised intervention he may make a referral for specialist help. Drugs do exist which are prescribed to people for depression. We feel that psychological interventions may be best tried first, particularly since some of the antidepressant medications used may decrease seizure threshold, thereby increasing the risk of fits. In addition, if a person can learn ways to overcome feelings of depression on his own, this will increase feelings of control and help him to cope in the future should such feelings arise again, as they are likely to do for most of us.

AGGRESSION AND DIFFICULT BEHAVIOUR

At one time, a commonly held belief was that people with epilepsy had a certain personality. Irritability, argumentativeness and even verbal and physical aggression were considered prominent features of the 'epileptic'. Descriptive phrases of this personality written in the early half of the twentieth century include 'over-sensitive', 'rigid', 'insistent on having one's own way', 'resentful of any interference' and 'self-centred'. Fortunately, evidence from research studies has not supported the existence of such a personality. It is true that some people with epilepsy can and do behave in this way, but so do a lot of people without epilepsy.

Aggressive behaviour as a feature of a fit is very rare and such behaviour would be expected to be short-lived and rather purposeless. A person may knock something over, break something, or knock into somebody during a fit, but this will be unintentional. Misunderstandings about a motive may arise if an individual experiences a period of confusion after a fit, with people trying to intervene too soon when he or she has not really come round. The person with epilepsy may then become agitated and perhaps verbally aggressive. If individuals have a good understanding of their epilepsy then they will know whether they experience such post-seizure states. If this has been identified, it can be conveyed to people when fits are described and this may reduce the likelihood of misunderstandings.

Rarely, antiepileptic drugs may make people irritable and less tolerant of situations. People with epilepsy will probably recognise this by experiencing a change in their ability to cope, in association with or shortly after a change in medication. People with epilepsy are the best ones to monitor their own behaviour, and if they feel such a change is taking place they should notify their doctor.

Epilepsy occurs in some people because of substantial damage to the brain. This is the case in only a minority of individuals; however, brain damage has been associated with difficult behaviour. The damaged brain means that the individual has fewer resources to be able to cope appropriately with frustration. They may also have difficulty expressing themselves verbally and making their concerns understood. Difficult behaviour may be encountered in individuals with brain damage whether or not they have seizures.

In the main, if people with epilepsy find themselves being irritable and aggressive, or feel that people are describing them in this way, the question 'Why?' must be asked. All too easily, people blame their epilepsy and their drugs. Sometimes irritability may be an indication the person is depressed. Understandably, having epilepsy may at times make people feel frustrated and annoyed. Why them, why not somebody else? It can be difficult to cope with the unpredictability of attacks. When people find they are feeling hostile and resentful, they must try to find out why and do something about such feelings. If they do not, other people will detect this antagonism and they may well lose friends.

A useful and simple way to begin to understand difficult

behaviour is to keep an anger diary. People should record angry feelings and outbursts, with details such as the time of day at which they occurred, where they were when it happened, what they were doing and who they were with. Keeping a diary every evening, say over a two-week period, can be quite revealing about factors underlying a person's anger. If people with epilepsy find they are continually feeling irritable and are over-reacting to small, silly events, they may benefit from relaxation exercises such as those mentioned earlier. They must be encouraged to look more closely at the way they cope with frustration, and perhaps to look for more appropriate ways of responding. Work may be needed on negative thoughts, learning to become aware when they are getting angry and trying to stay calm.

COGNITIVE DEFICITS

Cognitive function is a term used to refer to those processes whereby we take in information about the world around us, try to make sense of it, and act upon it. The term is used to cover such processes as the ability to concentrate on tasks, learning and memory, the ability to plan ahead and make decisions, and the ability to understand and express ourselves in language.

The brain is the place where cognitive function takes place. Research evidence has shown that different parts of our brain have slightly different roles. For example, for most people the left-hand side of the brain is important for processing verbal information, whereas the right-hand side is more important for processing visual and spatial information. Within each half of our brain different areas also seem to have specialist roles. For example, the temporal lobes of our brain are important for efficient memory. The left temporal lobe is generally considered important for verbal memory – things like learning people's names, learning new words, and written material for exams. The right temporal lobe is important for non-verbal memory – things like recognising people's faces and learning the way around new places. When the brain is not working properly, disorders of these functions can occur. However, for most people with epilepsy, the brain 'goes wrong' only rarely between attacks, and people are unlikely to experience significant problems.

Psychologists have developed special tests to measure different cognitive functions. The most well-known are measures of intelligence. These tests were developed primarily to predict how well children will do at school, and accordingly they tend to test skills valued in the education system, for example, verbal reasoning, knowledge of words and mathematical skills. Generally, intelligence tests are made up of various sub-tests and the overall score is usually expressed as an intelligence quotient (IQ). Most people will have IQ scores that fall in the average range, and this will be expressed as a figure between 90 and 109. Fewer people will have IQ scores that fall below average (less than 90) or above average (scores of 110 or more). Research studies have shown that most people with epilepsy also have IQ scores within the average range. There will also be a group of people with epilepsy who have above average intelligence and a group of people whose intelligence falls below average. Individuals in this latter group will include those with a mental handicap. Such individuals have limited ability as a result of a brain that is not functioning properly and generally this damage has existed from birth. The limited ability of these people is a reflection of their underlying brain damage, and is not a result of epilepsy. The association of mental handicap and epilepsy has wrongly led some people to believe that having epilepsy means a person will have low intelligence.

Families with a member who has epilepsy can often be concerned that the seizures will result in mental deterioration. Existing research evidence suggests that having fits is only rarely associated with such deterioration. In these cases it is often the result of an underlying degenerative disease, or else frequent status epilepticus may have occurred. These conditions happen only rarely. Improvements in treatment have occurred and medical intervention can very often prevent status epilepticus.

It is important to emphasise that intelligence tests do not measure all aspects of cognitive ability. For instance, many intelligence tests do not adequately measure important functions such as memory. To adequately assess such functions additional tests may be useful. An IQ figure, therefore, should not be given too much importance, or be taken out of context. There is increasing awareness that when considering a person's future prospects, other aspects of behaviour are equally important. For example, an individual's ability to get on with others may be as important as his or her IQ when considering suitability for a particular job.

Generally, epilepsy should not give rise to any specific cognitive difficulties. However, if people feel they are experiencing memory problems, or feel slowed down, or are having difficulty concentrating, this should be raised with their doctor. If many difficulties are felt to exist, they could be referred for a psychological assessment. This will involve them undertaking a series of special tests designed to measure different aspects of cognitive functioning. A thorough assessment may throw light on the nature of the difficulties, and may result in advice as to how these may affect various daily activities. Even more important, it may result in suggestions for ways to minimise these problems. If it was felt that medication was in any way implicated, a thorough assessment could be undertaken following changes in drug treatment.

Memory

Complaints of poor memory are probably the commonest problem reported by people with epilepsy. If people have complex partial seizures (which are originating from the temporal lobe), this may indeed result in an inefficient memory. It is the temporal lobe which is important for memory, as already mentioned. It has to be acknowledged that having epilepsy probably places more demands upon memory than other people might experience. People with epilepsy have a lot to remember – for example to take their tablets at specific times, to keep appointments, and often to keep detailed accounts of their seizures for presentation at clinic visits. It is possible that medication for epilepsy may influence memory. Decreasing medication, however, may have the unwanted effect of an increase in seizures, which is equally undesirable. Memory difficulties seldom disappear completely following a change in medication, and there are no drugs in existence to improve memory – a memory-improving pill would be a nice easy solution, but unfortunately none exists. Some people with epilepsy may have to accept that they will have to live with a poor memory. The first step to coping with a memory difficulty is actually knowing that one exists. It is then possible to take precautions to get around any potential problems. People should also be aware that mood can influence memory. When people are anxious and depressed, their memory is likely to be unreliable.

Internal strategies	External strategies

visual imagery:
  names
  peg methods
  methods of loci
verbal methods:
  stories
  rhymes
  first letter techniques
	lists
	memory boards
	diaries
	alarm clocks and watches
	memory aid calculators
	drug wallets

The table above gives a list of strategies that may support a weak memory. They are divided into two main groups: internal and external measures. The former are the ones widely recommended by advertisements which appear in newspapers to 'improve your memory'. They can be useful, but only when the amount that has to be remembered is quite limited. Visual imagery is applied to techniques where individuals make mental pictures involving the information to be remembered. Some people are much better at doing this than others. It can be helpful for remembering a few important names – for example, a bizarre image can be made in association with a name. The best way of using these methods is for people to try to incorporate a distinctive feature of the person into their image. For example, if the person is called Mr Herring and has a rather prominent nose then an image incorporating a long nose on a fish may be successful (*see* Fig 7). Of course, this can be very difficult with some names – for example, thinking of a mental image for a Mrs Jones or a Dr Smythe.

Peg-type strategies (Fig 8) involve learning a set of standard words, often in the form of a poem. A commonly reported one is of the format: one is a bun, two is a shoe, three is a tree, four is a door, five is a hive, and so on. Having learned this group of words, it may be possible for people to use it to help them remember things. For example, on a particular day a person may have to remember to

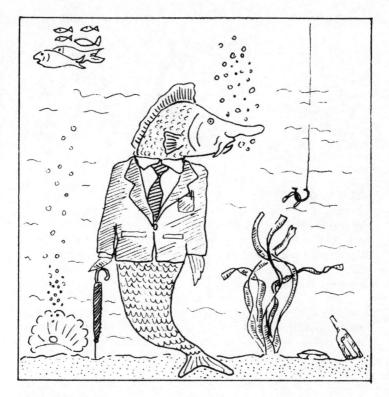

Fig 7 Mr Herring.

post a letter, phone the dentist to cancel an appointment, and collect their clothes from the cleaners. Using the peg-type strategy they would first of all make a bizarre image incorporating 'one is a bun' by perhaps imagining a bun with a letter-box in it and a letter poking out. They could use 'two is a shoe' to remember to phone the dentist by imagining a shoe with very large teeth like an open mouth, with a telephone by the side. To remember to collect the clothes from the cleaners, they would use 'three is a tree' – perhaps by imagining their clothes hanging from a tree (*see* Fig 8).

A similar strategy is the method of loci. In this, items to be remembered are associated with a particular location, perhaps the rooms in a house or places on a commonly taken walk or journey. People could perhaps begin with the kitchen and imagine a letter

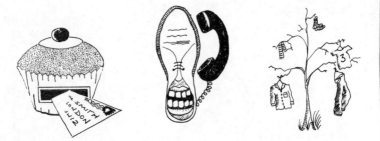

Fig 8   Peg-type strategy.

popping out of the toaster. The next thing to remember is to phone the dentist, and the person might imagine walking into the lounge and looking out of the window which has been transformed into a large gaping mouth with prominent teeth. Finally, to remember the clothes, one could imagine walking up the stairs with clothes scattered around (*see* Fig 9).

There are a number of verbal memory aids which some people find useful – for example, simply making up a story about all the activities to be remembered or turning them into a short poem. Many people may have come across this strategy, especially at school when learning the number of days in the month by the rhyme, 'Thirty days has September, April, June and November...' and so on. The 'first letter' technique is also familiar to most people, and many children have learned the colours of the rainbow by remembering the sentence, 'Richard Of York Gave Battle In Vain'.

External memory strategies are the most widely used. They can be divided into techniques to aid information storage, and cueing devices which help to prompt people to do things. Shopping lists and memory boards can be useful. Many people with or without epilepsy become dependent on their diaries for the activities they have to carry out each day. Diaries can be very helpful, particularly if a person looks at them every morning. There is a whole range of information that it would be impossible for us to keep in our heads, such as details of bank accounts, people's birthdays, telephone numbers and so on, which can be stored in this way.

A knot in the handkerchief is commonly thought of as a cueing aid; however, its effectiveness has been questioned. It reminds us that we had something to remember but it tells us nothing about

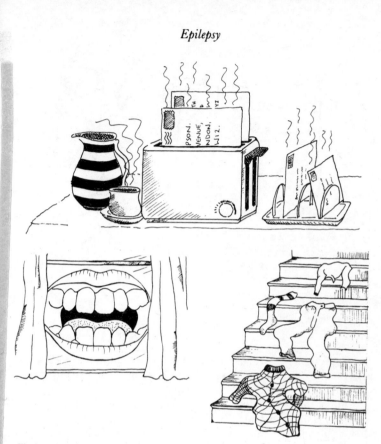

Fig 9   Method of loci.

what it was we have to recall. Other types of cueing device include
alarm clocks which can be set at certain times, perhaps the time
when the person has to take some medication. Digital watches now
often have alarm devices that can be set to go off at certain intervals.
There are also a growing number of commercially available cueing
devices such as electronic diaries. These generally consist of a system
like an alarm clock and a pad of paper. Each page is divided into
days and times. A person jots down in advance something which
needs to be done at a particular time, and sets the alarm. When the
alarm goes off, a glance at the diary indicates what has to be
remembered. Some electronic calculators also exist which have

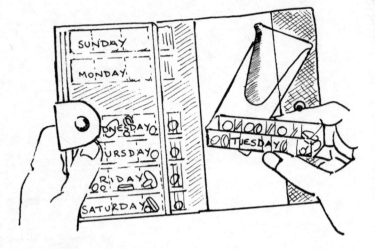

Fig 10 A drug wallet.

alarm functions which can be set to the minute, and some calculators can be programmed not only to ring an alarm but also to give a cue as to what has to be remembered.

One of the most valuable external memory aids for people with epilepsy is the drug wallet (*see* Fig 10). Many people find this device helps them to remember to take their tablets, and also not to take too many. The drug wallets available usually consist of seven small containers, one for each day of the week. Each container is divided into sections generally marked morning, afternoon and evening. The compartments can be filled once a week at set regular times. The seven individual containers are removable, so that if a person goes out for the day they do not have to take the complete set, which is rather bulky. Drug wallets can be obtained from local chemists, and are not too expensive.

Another suggestion which we would make for people with epilepsy is to make notes before a visit to the doctor about the things that are of concern and the issues that need clarifying. It may also be useful to note down things which are said during the interview for future reference.

Glossary

Automatism   During complex partial seizures, people may sometimes do things in a state of diminished awareness, for instance plucking at their clothes, fiddling with various objects, making lip-smacking or chewing movements, grimacing, undressing, performing aimless activities, or wandering around in a confused fashion.

Aura   People with partial epilepsy may sometimes get a warning of an impending fit, which is called the aura. This means that the seizure has a simple partial onset. What actually happens in the aura depends on the area of the brain in which the epileptic discharge starts.

Automatic behaviour   *see* Automatism.

Brain stem   The part of the brain situated between the cerebrum and the spinal cord. It could be described as the main switchboard of the brain. It is responsible for many of the functions of the body which happen independently of one's will – for example, breathing, sleep and digestion.

Cerebellum   Part of the brain which controls co-ordination and balance. It is situated in the back of the brain and is about the size of an apple.

Cerebrospinal fluid   Watery liquid which circulates around the brain, with functions similar to the blood. Examination of the cerebrospinal fluid is sometimes needed to rule out certain diseases, especially infections.

Corticosteroids   Powerful drugs widely used in several fields of medicine. They are synthetic forms of a hormone produced by the adrenal gland.

Cryptogenic   Condition or disease for which no cause is known.

Cyanosis   A bluish or purplish discoloration of the skin due to lack of oxygen in the blood.

Focus   An epileptic focus is the part of the brain in which an epileptic discharge starts.

Glaucoma   A disease of the eye in which the internal pressure of the eye is increased.

Haemorrhage   Loss of blood from a vessel; bleeding.

Idiopathic   *see* Cryptogenic.

Meninges   Special tissue which covers the brain and spinal cord.

Meningitis   Infection of the meninges.

Migraine   A form of one sided headache which happens intermittently, often accompanied by nausea and disorders of vision. Other signs of temporary brain malfunction may occasionally occur.

Neurofibromatosis   A hereditary disease characterised by small lumps on the skin, brown-coloured skin spots, and which sometimes may be associated with benign brain tumours, which may cause epilepsy.

Paroxysms   Short-lived intermittent episodes.

Spasticity   A condition in which the muscles in a particular part of the body are tightened.

Stroke   Symptoms and signs brought about by a sudden interruption of the blood supply to a part of the brain or in a few cases by a bleed in the brain (brain haemorrhage). The most common cause for a stroke is a blood clot blocking a vessel, thus causing an interruption of the blood supply.

Symptomatic   Describes a condition for which a cause is known, as opposed to a cryptogenic condition, for which no cause is known or found.

Syndrome   A set of signs and symptoms which, when taken together, make up the picture of a disease.

Trigeminal neuralgia   Intermittent facial pain, also known as 'tic doloreux'.

Tuberous sclerosis   A condition, usually hereditary, which presents with skin abnormalities and calcifications in the brain of the people affected. It may be a cause of epilepsy and mental retardation.

Further Reading

About epilepsy

Aspinall, A. and Jeavons, P., *Epilepsy Reference Book*, Harper and Row, 1985

Chadwick, D. and Usiskin, S., *Living with Epilepsy*, Macdonald, 1987

Laidlaw, J. and Laidlaw, M., *Epilepsy Explained*, Churchill-Livingstone, 1980

McGoven, S., *The Epilepsy Handbook*, Sheldon Press, 1982

About psychological problems

Blackburn, I. M., *Coping with Depression*, Chambers, 1987

Macdonald Wallace, J., *Stress – A Practical Guide to Coping*, The Crowood Press, 1988

Whitmore, B., *Living with Stress and Anxiety*, Manchester University Press, 1987

Useful Addresses

Assessment Centres for Epilepsy

Bootham Park Hospital
Bootham
York
YO3 7BY
Tel: 0904 54664

Chalfont Centre for Epilepsy
Chalfont St. Peter
Buckinghamshire
SL9 0RJ
Tel: 024 07 3991

David Lewis Centre*
Alderley Edge
Mobberley
Cheshire
SK9 7UD
Tel: 056 587 2613

Maudsley Hospital – Epilepsy
   Unit*
Denmark Hill
London
SE5 8AZ
Tel: 01 703 6333

Park Hospital for Children
Oxford
OX3 7LQ
Tel: 0865 245651

* Not designated special
assessment centres, but
provide an assessment facility
for people with epilepsy.

National Voluntary Organisations

British Epilepsy Association
Anstey House
40 Hanover Square
Leeds
LS3 1BE
for membership enquiries
Tel: 0532 439393
for general information
Tel: 0345 089599
Regional offices:
London   *Tel*: 01 929 4069
Belfast   *Tel*: 0232 248414

Epilepsy Association of
   Scotland [Glasgow]
48 Govan Road
Glasgow
G51 1JR
Tel: 041 427 4911

Epilepsy Association for
    Scotland [Edinburgh]
13 Guthrie Street
Edinburgh
EH1 1JG
Tel: 031 226 5458

Irish Epilepsy Association
249 Crumlin Road
Dublin W12
Tel: 01 557500

National Society for Epilepsy
Chalfont Centre for Epilepsy
Chalfont St. Peter
Buckinghamshire
SL9 0RJ
Tel: 024 07 3991

Wales Epilepsy Association
Gwynedd Voluntary Services
    Council
Eldon Square
Dolgellau
Gwynedd
Tel: 0341 422575

Special Schools for Children with Epilepsy

David Lewis Centre
Alderley Edge
Mobberley
Cheshire
SK9 7UD
Tel: 056 587 2613

Lingfield Hospital School
Lingfield
Surrey
RH7 6PN
Tel: 0342 832243

St. Elizabeth's School
Much Hadham
Hertfordshire
SG10 6EW
Tel: 027 984 3451

Medic-Alert Foundation

Medic-Alert Foundation
11/13 Clifton Terrace
London
N4 3JP
Tel: 01 263 8596

Index